LOW BACK PAIN

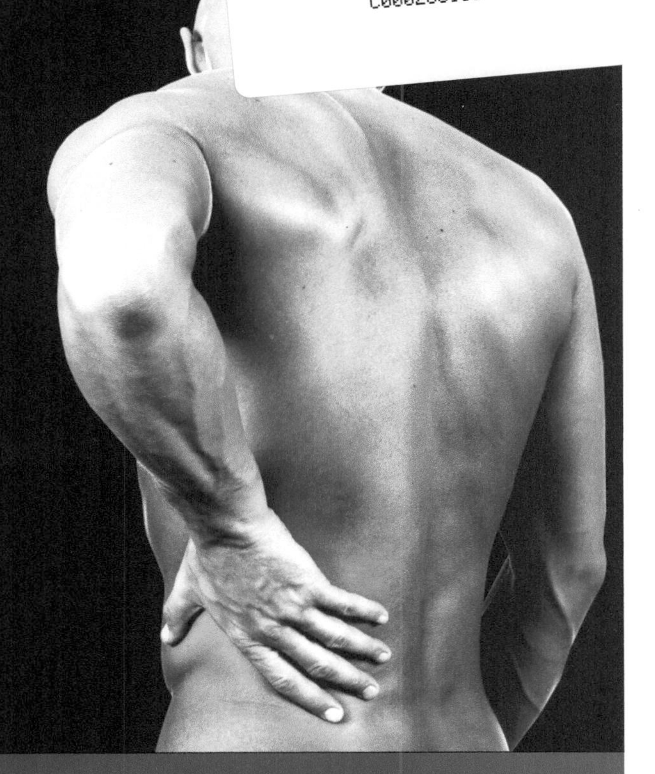

What patients and primary health care providers should know.

REY LAZARO, M.D.

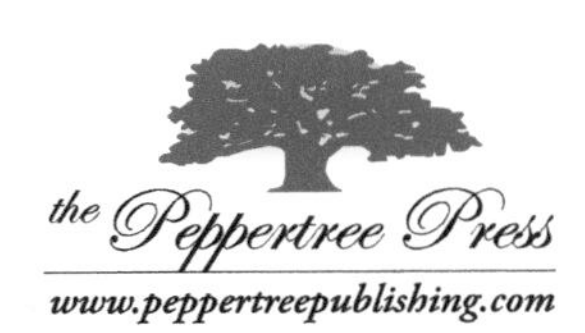

Also written by Rey Lazaro, M.D.

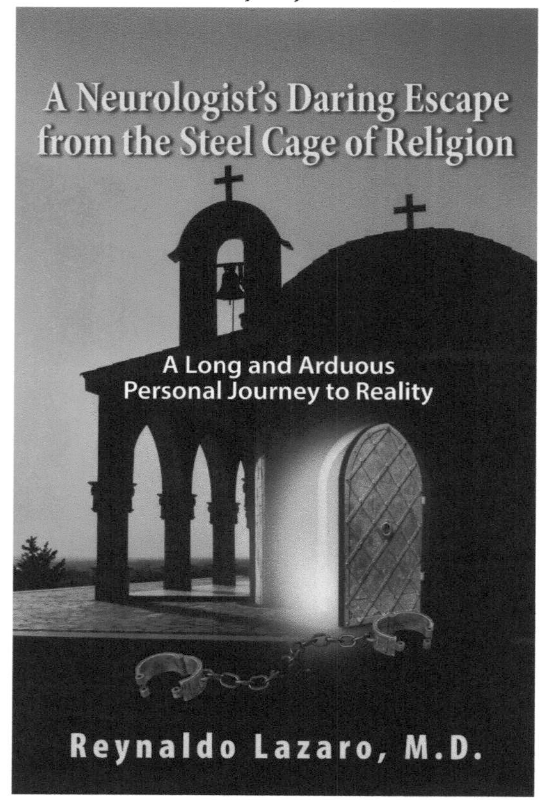

 Graphic design by: Elizabeth Parry

For information regarding permission, call 941-922-2662 or contact us at our website: www.peppertreepublishing.com or write to: The Peppertree Press, LLC. Attention: Publisher 715 N. Washington Blvd., Suite B, Sarasota, Florida 34236

ISBN: 978-1-61493-842-2
Library of Congress: 2022914304
Printed: August 2022

DEDICATION

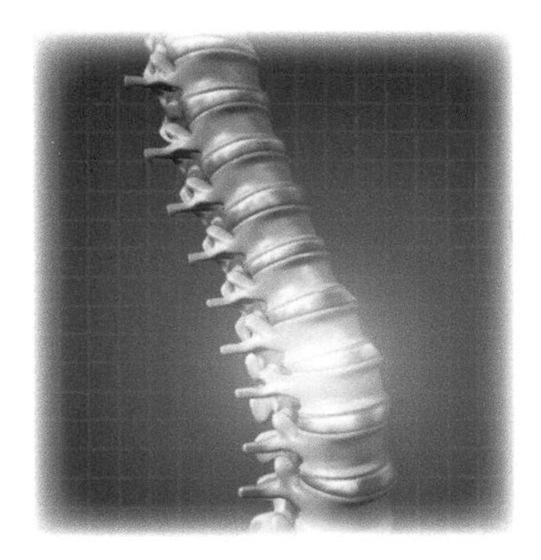

This book is dedicated to all low back pain sufferers who became permanently incapacitated despite receiving numerous conservative and interventional therapies, and to several healthcare providers who put their trust in me to provide them with much-needed neurological information.

Allow me to picture a scenario on how we might have gotten to get the way we are now – erect! One day… trying to pick some hard-to-reach fruit from some overhanging branches, one creative ancestor of ours tried "standing" on his two hind limbs. Then with the two front ones, started picking the fruit which he could otherwise not get to. And just like that, the evolutionary process began to slowly take place. Now, being upright we put a lot more stress on that back – the lower back particularly. Alas… that miserable low back pain.—Dr. Alfredo I. Custodio, *You've Got M@il,* Palmetto, 2021.

INTRODUCTION

"Dear back pain, please go. I can't stand, neither sit nor bow!!"

"87% of young people have back pain. The other 13% have no computer."

"Technically, I'm still young but according to my back pain, I'm actually 97."

– *www.therandomvibes.com/back-pain-quotes*

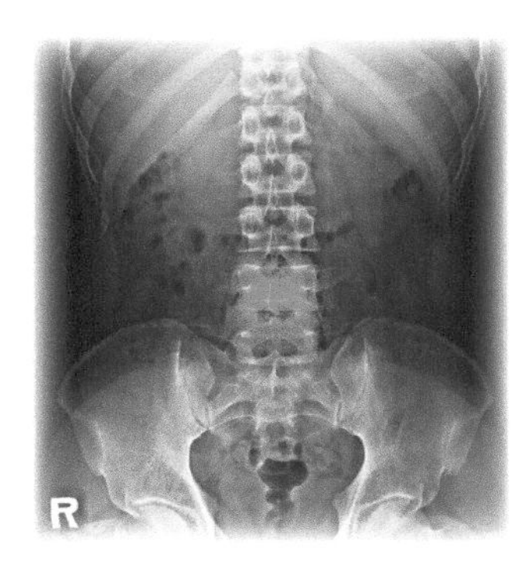

The lumbar spine is a complex biological pillar, embryologically well-engineered, multi-articular, and multifaceted superstructure that connects with and supports the upper half of the body. This part of the spine provides an extensive nerve supply to the lower extremities, including the nerves that control the urinary bladder and anal muscles. It is always mechanically active, and under stress most of the time, regardless of body position–whether standing, sitting, and lying down—and, depending on the nature of the stress exerted against it, pain may occur transiently or recur and could become chronically debilitating and emotionally draining. Pain can generate or arise from different structures and articulations, and it varies in severity and duration. It can be localized and diffuse, or it can extend down to the lower extremity, unilaterally or bilaterally, and may, in some cases, be associated with symptoms such as "pins and needles" (paresthesias), numbness, cold or warm sensations, cramps, and muscle weakness.

Low back pain (LBP) is a frequent complaint that brings patients to their healthcare providers. The type of pain can be acute, chronic, or recurrent, with remissions and exacerbations. Causative factors are non-occupational or occupational, and some are related to vehicular or sports accident injuries. Some cases develop in association with systemic diseases and malignancy, and some are due to genetic factors. Aging is a common risk factor. Moreover, more than one structure in the spinal column may contribute to the pain at any one time, although they are frequently indistinguishable from each other. Healthcare costs incurred from various diagnostic procedures, treatment modalities, and legal proceedings can put tremendous strain on the finances of patients and insurance companies.[45,50] Persistent pain and treatment failures frequently lead to mental anguish, depression, and long-term disability, not to mention drug dependence or an addiction to narcotic analgesics.

Diagnostic test procedures utilized for LBP include plain x-rays, computerized axial tomography (CAT) scans, magnetic resonance imaging (MRI), electromyography (EMG), thermal imaging, bone scans, single proton emission computed tomography (SPECT), ultrasound, discography, and myelography. [4,26,29,33,48,64,69,74,84,94,100,109] For a great majority of LBP sufferers, not all of these tests are necessary. Some are harmless and painless, some are uncomfortable, and some, particularly EMG and discography, can be quite painful. Radiation exposure from plain x-rays, CAT scans, bone scans, and SPECT is minimal as long as the procedure is performed infrequently. Myelography can produce transient systemic and allergic reactions, vomiting, and dizziness. Infection, although rare, can occur. Postural headache—a type of headache that exacerbates when standing and recedes when lying down—resulting from a spinal fluid leak secondary to a lumbar puncture can occur in some situations and may require an epidural blood patch to plug the punctured site.

The treatment approach for LBP varies depending on the anatomical location of the generator of pain and the presence or absence of neurological deficits. The necessity for accurate localization of the generator of pain is a crucial factor in failed low back surgery syndrome (FLBSS).[2,6,15,19.23,40,68,88,97] There are several treatment modalities for LBP that are either conservative or invasive. The former consists of analgesics, anti-inflammatory medications, rest, physical exercise, and spinal adjustments, while the latter consists of various forms of spinal injections and surgical interventions. Other alternative therapies include acupuncture, biofeedback, and the intake of herbal products. Transcutaneous nerve stimulation devices and spinal cord stimulators have also been used in FBLSS and persistent intractable pain with variable results, as well as several adverse side effects and complications.

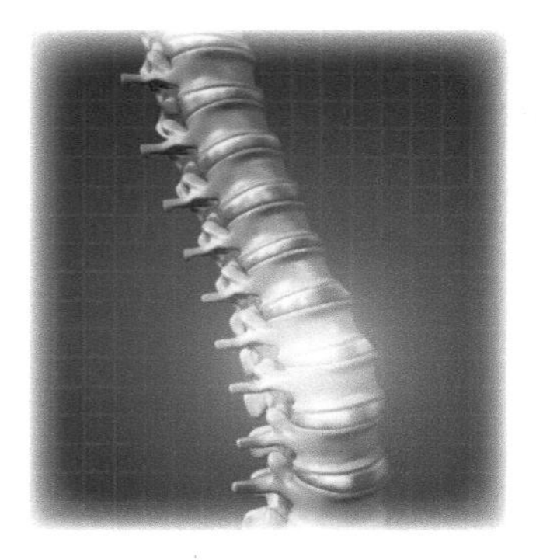

It is of paramount importance to make patients aware that the success of treatment depends highly on the recognition of the presence or absence of symptoms that accompany LBP and the identification of the nature or location of the generator of pain through the use of certain diagnostic procedures. Patients should be informed of the accuracy of certain diagnostic procedures and how they affect the function for which they are being used. However, based on my experience, this information is almost always unavailable to patients at the time of the initial neurologic consultation for a variety of reason, one of which is lack of communication between the health care provider and the patient. This is unfortunate because it can be disconcerting for patients to be informed that the results of a test procedure are normal or mildly abnormal in the presence of severe LBP. Conversely, an abnormal test result does not necessarily identify the precise source or cause of the symptoms. Such a scenario is not only an invitation for treatment failure and an unhappy patient who is suffering physically and mentally, but it can also lead to medical and legal controversies.

In most surgical clinics, the decision to operate is left to the surgical team after all the results of the diagnostic procedures have been made available. In some situations, the surgeon may be pressured to operate despite a lack of clear correlation between the laboratory and clinical presentation, especially when a desperate patient is in severe and unrelenting pain. Clinicians, particularly neurologists, are not usually asked to participate in the decision-making process, except when they are requested to perform a clinical consultation and/or electromyographic examination. In my opinion, the decision-making process must be a team effort, and that means inviting a neurologist (and other specialists) with expertise in peripheral neurology or neuromuscular disorders to join the team and to actively participate in the discussion of such important and delicate issues in the care of patients with LBP being considered for possible surgery. Such an approach can have a positive and favorable effect on the patient–physician relationship.

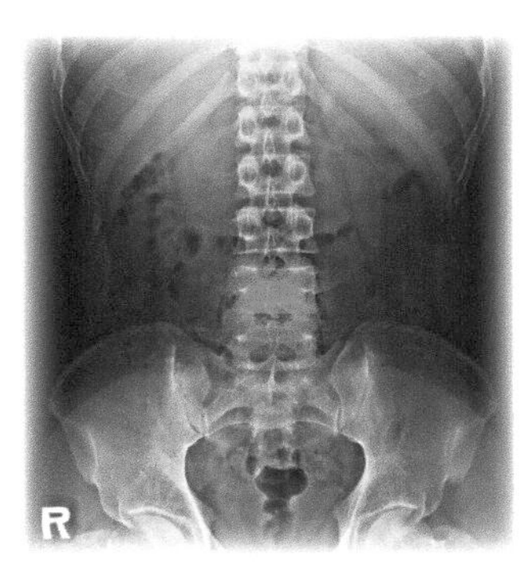

It still appalls me to this day that the presence of a herniated or bulging disk is frequently construed as the cause of LBP and that correcting the displaced disk can eliminate the pain. In reality, and not uncommonly, this is not the case. I will discuss this matter in Chapter 7, together with the utility, accuracy, and sensitivity of some diagnostic procedures. Misleading information and results obtained from these procedures, along with medical and legal ramifications, are also discussed in the Chapter.

The comments and opinions I present and discuss in this book are based on fifty years of experience as a neurologist with expertise in neuromuscular disorders. This experience is corroborated by voluminous literature and articles (including my own) written by various national and international medical and surgical experts, which are listed in the bibliography. I discuss some topics in great and revealing detail, but others only superficially—my apologies for the latter, but I have attempted to cite as many references as possible for readers to search to satisfy their curiosity and inquiring minds. There are several medical terms used in this book that some laypersons who happen to have the time to read this book may find disconcerting or upsetting. Again, please accept my apologies. However, in modern times, one click on your computer's electronic "rodent" using your index finger will provide a quick answer to your queries. I have repeated some remarks a few times during the course of discussing certain topics, but this was done on purpose to make and stress a point.

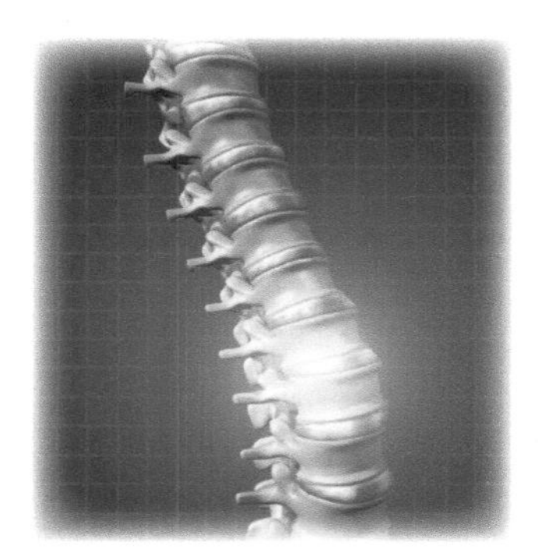

ACKNOWLEDGMENTS

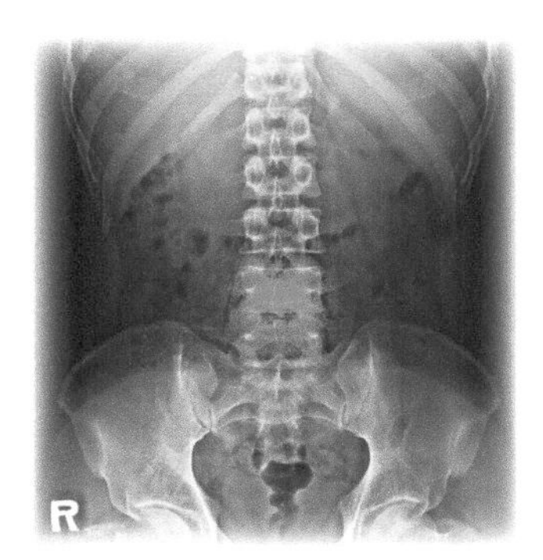

I thank the several hundreds of patients (me included) whom I have evaluated over the past forty-five years for the encouragement they gave me to write this book. The pain they endured even after the institution of various treatment modalities—conservative and interventional—provided the impetus for me to "spill the beans" and provide a reasonable scientific explanation for the persistence of their pain. My even-tempered and understanding roommate of fifty-two years, Zeny, continues to willingly and unselfishly provide me with much-needed high-octane inspiration to keep the axoplasm of my cerebral neurons revving up and flowing smoothly. Without this fuel, this piece of work would have been incomplete, disorganized, and buried under a foot of dust in my library. My classmate, Dr. Alfredo I. Custodio, a physician writer, a successful surgeon in the "Show Me" State of Missouri, and the chief of the Grammar Police Force of the 1970 medical alumni e-mail group, provided strong words of encouragement.

ABOUT THE AUTHOR

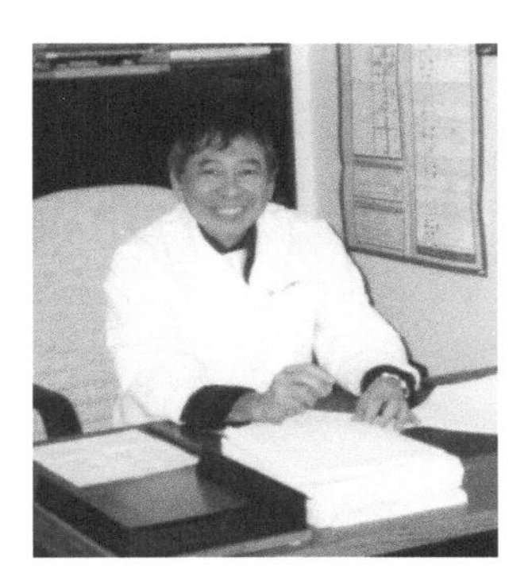

Dr. Rey Lazaro resides in Guilderland, a small quiet town in Upstate New York, west of Albany. A graduate of the University of Santo Tomas Faculty of Medicine and Surgery in Manila, Philippines in 1970, he received his training in neurology at St. Vincent Hospital and Medical Center of New York, and his training in neuromuscular disorders and electromyography at Vanderbilt University Medical Center in Nashville, Tennessee. He is board-certified in adult neurology and electrodiagnostic medicine. During his fifty-plus years of practice, he evaluated numerous patients who sustained job-related and vehicular-accident-related injuries. He spends most of his time in semi-retirement doing clinical research. He has published numerous scientific articles on hereditary and acquired neuromuscular disorders, electromyography, low back pain, radiculopathies, and entrapment neuropathies.

TABLE OF CONTENTS

CHAPTER 1

Brief Historical Background, Primate-to-Man Evolution, Genetics, and Biomechanics of the Lumbar Spine

We are the product of 4.5 billion years of fortuitous, slow biological evolution. There is no reason to think that the evolutionary process has stopped. Man is a transitional animal. He is not the climax of creation.

—Carl Sagan (1934–1996), American astrophysicist, cosmologist, and science educator.

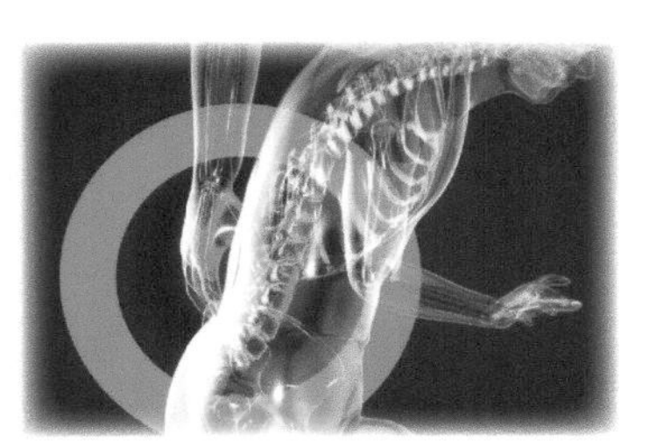

The inordinately high incidence of low back pain (LBP) among modern humans is putatively linked to the evolutionary process in the primate family tree—from quadrupedal to bipedal locomotion. When humans began walking upright, the mechanical forces exerted on the articulations and ligaments that held the vertebral bodies stacked together in the spinal column increased. Unique to the erect human spine are the lateral spinal ligaments, which are absent in quadrupeds.[54] The development of these ligaments along with the interspinous and supraspinous, anterior and posterior, longitudinal and capsular ligaments are fundamental to the mechanical stability of an erect spine, enabling it to be both flexible and stable—in contrast to the relatively rigid lumbar spine of quadrupeds.[54] The flexibility and stability are further enhanced and reinforced by various paraspinal muscles. However, the present modern-day living conditions, involving protracted sitting and leaning over on the work desk, long interstate highway driving, highly strenuous activities in construction and agriculture, and any type of occupation that leads to poor posture, are contributory factors to the development of disk degeneration.

The centerpiece of the vertebral column, which is commonly equated with LBP, is the disk composed of several layers of tough collagen protein fibers (annulus fibrosus) and softer collagen protein located in the center (nucleus pulposus). Each disk has upper and lower surfaces attached to the vertebral endplate, which consist of cortical bone and hyaline cartilage. Mechanically, the disk is the main shock absorber or cushion that protects the vertebra above and below from rubbing against each other. Flexibility decreases with age as it becomes calcified or dehydrated (the nucleus pulposus contains 70%–90% water). High-pressure vertical forces, such as prolonged sitting or standing and unsupported bending, can displace the disk centrally or laterally. A displaced disk, seen frequently at L4–5 and L5S1, is called bulging or protruding and, when displaced significantly, is called a herniated nucleus pulposus or herniated disk (HD). The process of disk degeneration involves loss of water content followed by calcification, resulting in narrowing of the intervertebral space. This degenerative process is frequently implicated in LBP, and typically starts after age 40. The normal adult disk is relatively avascular, and it relies on diffusion for its supply of nutrients.

Intervertebral disk disease (IDD) is also common among quadrupeds, such as canines and felines, which have a pathology similar to that of humans. Among dogs, neurologic deficits resulting from IDD are common, especially when the disk herniates (10). Axial compression stress is greater in dogs than in humans owing to higher vertebral densities. In addition, the thickness of the ligaments in the ventral and dorsal parts of the annulus fibrosus is uneven, and the rotation is limited by the facet joints, which play a role in stabilizing the spine during running and jumping. During the process of disk degeneration, lumbar disk herniation is likely to occur. In dogs, spinal cord compression becomes inevitable because the cord terminates between the last two vertebrae (L6–L7) compared to L1–L2 in humans, and below this level, nerve roots and/or cauda equina will likely be affected. Such an event tends to cause paralysis and bladder disturbances.

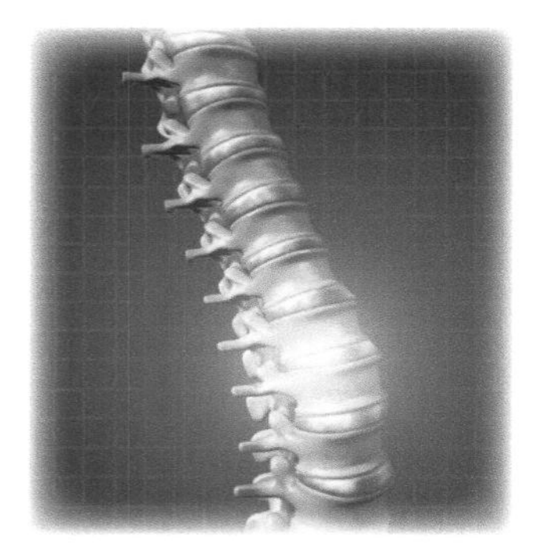

There is another side of the story that needs to be told to laypersons concerning the biomechanical forces exerted on the disks and spinal articulations that take place in humans during the slow and nebulous process of evolution, from quadrupedal to bipedal locomotion. If there is such a thing as evolution, it must be explained more deeply at the molecular and genetic levels. Superficially, the way evolution is being taught and explained in the media outlet and periodicals is quite simplistic, but most erudite skeptics have a different take and a more in-depth elucidation of this subject. An analogy can be made with religious indoctrination propagated through belief systems by the ancients, who at that time possessed no scientific knowledge or sophisticated equipment to document and provide hard copies of certain miraculous or historical events. Owing to our present understanding of biochemistry and the molecular basis of life, If evolution is to be believed and authenticated, it must be accomplished by investigating and documenting the alterations that take place in the structure of primate and human chromosomes. Therefore, evolution should be defined in the context of molecular alteration or restructuring of the gene content of the family tree of primates.

Humans have forty-six chromosomes, and apes have forty-eight. While some parts of the human and ape chromosomes are similar, the genomes are vastly different, based on hard scientific evidence (105). The difference has been attributed to a fusion of the ends of two small, ape-like chromosomes in a human-ape ancestor that presumably occurred in the distant past and eventually formed human chromosome 2. This theory has since been debunked by some geneticists.[Online3-6] Nevertheless, this issue of the evolutionary process remains unresolved. Moreover, the Y chromosomes of chimpanzees and humans are remarkably divergent in structure and gene composition.[28,37,38,51] This difference is such that the "ape to human transition" is clearly untenable, according to some experts.[6] Moreover, the chimpanzee Y chromosome has thirty-seven genes, and the human has seventy-eight or more. The main issue now is that for evolution to proceed accordingly, it would require a monumental and colossal task for such a process to take place at a biomolecular level—a statistical and logistical improbability. How this all came about would depend on what side of the fence you are sitting on—intelligent intervention from a divine power or from advanced extraterrestrial involvement—or maybe from nebulous natural forces.[Book3-5] It says in the book of genesis, "And God said, let us make man in our image." Why did God speak in the plural? Were there "gods" from outer space (extra- or intraterrestial) that were responsible for the so-called evolution of primate chromosomes?

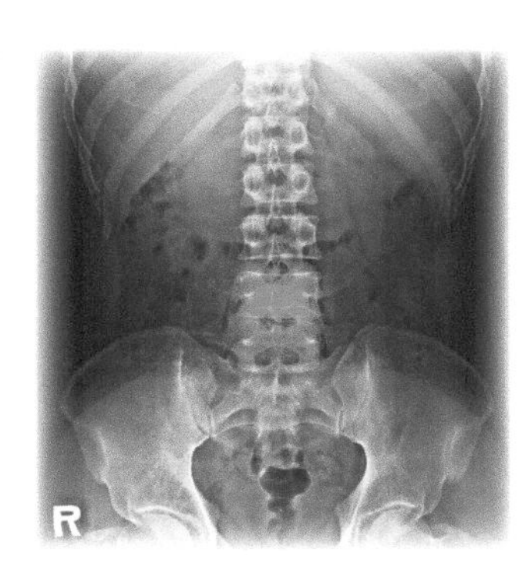

The foregoing discussion was not meant to deviate from the original theme of this book, but to serve as a prelude to various intriguing revelations that I discuss in the text—those that may change the perspective of laypersons and LBP sufferers. The opinions and views expressed in this piece of work were based on my fifty years of experience as a neurologist with expertise in neuromuscular disorders. During those years, I analyzed in great detail the nature and pattern of LBP and its associated symptoms and examined how they can predict the results of a diagnostic procedure or affect the outcome of a treatment modality, particularly surgery.

CHAPTER 2 Anatomy of the lumbar spine, neural innervations, sinuvertebral nerves, and blood supply

My life changed irrevocably four and a half years ago. I spent two years on the floor in excruciating, debilitating, and unrelenting pain. I can only describe the pain as being submerged into a vat of scalding acid that has an electric current running through it. And you can never get out, ever.

—Bill Walton, former great NBA basketball player

You know you're getting older when your back starts going out more than you do.

—Phyllis Diller (1917–2012), American actress and comedian

If the spine were a rigid and unyielding structure like a piece of solid metal rod, the dexterous and agile maneuverability—a functional necessity of the human lifestyle—would be greatly impaired, if not impossible, to perform. The spine is composed of several vertebrae (seven cervical, twelve thoracic, five lumbar, five sacral, and four coccygeal) stacked one on top of the other, supported by ligaments and tough fibrous tissues, and joined by several articular surfaces, including the disks located in between them, all of which are supplied by various pain-sensitive nerve fibers.[83] The paraspinal muscles, which are attached and surround the spine, help protect the spinal segments and maintain the proper posture and normal lordotic curve of the lumbar spine.[101] This arrangement makes the spine flexible yet stable. However, during the aging process or following the surgical fusion of two or more vertebrae, the spine becomes rigid and less flexible. The spine is made of thirty-three bony vertebrae extending from the base of the skull to the middle of the upper buttock. Enclosed within it is the spinal cord, which is an extension of the brain and brainstem extending from the top of the neck and down to the first (or second) lumbar vertebra. Inside the spinal cord are numerous nerve tracts that carry different motor and sensory fibers. The spine is the main "conduit" that connects the brain to the upper and lower extremities and trunk via various nerve roots and peripheral nerve bundles. Disorders or lesions of the cervical and thoracic spine will give rise to symptoms different from those located in the lumbar, sacral, and coccygeal segments of the spine because of the presence of the spinal cord above the lumbar spine. Therefore, the symptoms stemming from any lesions in the lumbar spine are due to the involvement of nerve roots and/or the cauda equina, not the spinal cord. The main focus of this book is on the lumbar spine.

The larger size of the lumbar vertebrae is understandable since it is the only bony and fibrocartilaginous structure that bears the brunt of full responsibility to support the upper half of the body. Of course, realistically speaking, the nerve roots and peripheral nerves originating from the lumbar spine control the sensory and motor function of the lower extremities together, including urogenital and anal physiology. In essence, the entire body is supported and controlled by the lumbar spine. The vertebral body and arches are the basic frames of each vertebra. Each arch consists of a pair of tough pedicles and laminae that form the wall of the vertebral foramen through which the spinal nerve passes. The lordotic angle of the vertebrae is attributed to the broader anterior segment creating the lumbosacral angle. Its natural design (similar to those in the cervical and thoracic spinal column) is somewhat rough and rugged because of the several protruding parts, which are medically termed "processes" (transverse, articular, spinous, accessory, and mammillary). Each process is attached to similar corresponding processes above and below each vertebra, and they are all held together by tough ligaments. Present throughout the spinal column are the posterior and anterior longitudinal ligaments and interspinous and supraspinous ligaments that connect the adjacent vertebra and spinous processes.[101]

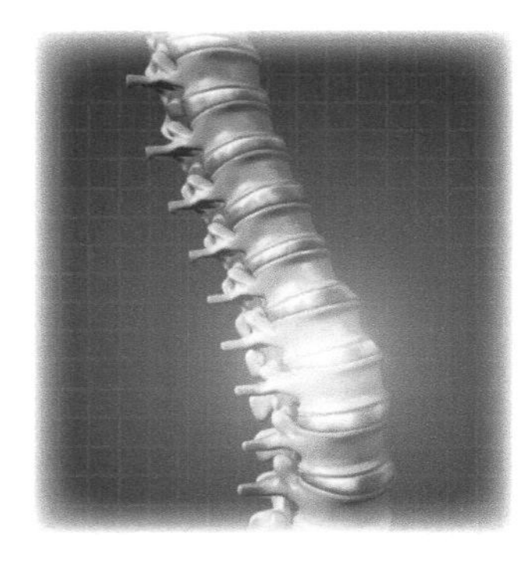

Between each vertebra are the disks. As discussed in Chapter 1, the disk consists of a ring of crisscrossing fibrous bands called the annulus fibrosus, and a gel-filled elastic central part known as nucleus pulposus. The fluid content changes with body position—during the night, and when lying in the supine position, the fluid retreats; it is then pushed out during the daytime and when an upright position. The disks are protected by the anterior and posterior longitudinal ligaments, which are wider and more adherent to the annulus fibrosus than the vertebral body. This anatomical arrangement is more prominent in the posterior longitudinal ligaments, where they appear much thinner, making it relevant to the pathogenesis of posterolateral disk herniations.

In the pathologic state, various degrees of bone marrow changes occur within the vertebral body, which can be seen clearly on an MRI.[31,85,120] These changes, which have been associated with LBP and degenerative disk disease, were first described by Dr. Michael T. Modic of Vanderbilt University Medical Center, who classified them into four types: Type 0—normal disk and vertebral body; Type 1—disruption and fissuring of the end plates and bone marrow edema, characterized by decreased signal on T1-weighted images and an increased signal intensity on T2-weighted images; Type 2—fatty replacement of the bone marrow within the vertebral body, characterized by increased signal intensity on both T1- and T2-weighted images; and Type 3—subchondral bone marrow sclerosis characterized by decreased signal intensity on both T1- and T2-weighted sequences. The precise correlation between these findings and clinical symptoms is not well defined, although it seems that a higher incidence of LBP is associated with Modic changes. Some think that Modic type 1 may represent an autoimmune response to the cells of the nucleus pulposus.

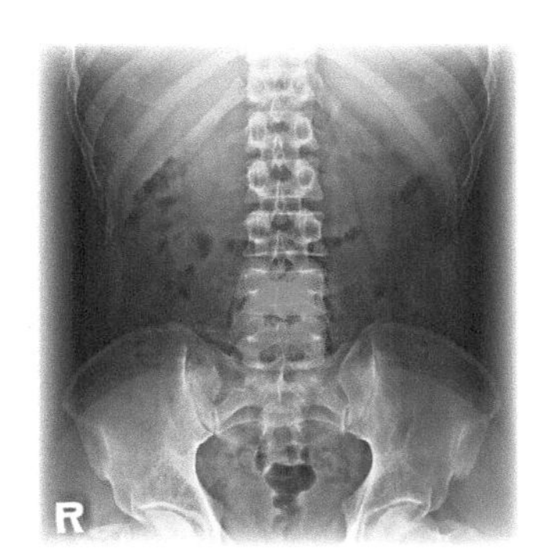

The articulations that are located at the back of each spinal segment, which have received more attention in recent years, are the two pairs of facet joints (or zygapophyseal joints) in each vertebra; one pair (superior facet joint) connects to the vertebra above, while the other pair (inferior facet joint) connects to the one below. Like the intervertebral disks, they bear a significant amount of stress in an upright position and are subject to degenerative process and injury. These joints are purported to be one of the main generators of LBP, particularly when the joints undergo degradation, as in osteoarthritis and spondylosis. They allow for various spinal movements, such as flexion and extension, and protect the spine from rotational injury. Pain usually originates from the cartilaginous capsule of the joints and is likely to occur when the synovial membrane ceases to secrete fluid, leading to friction between joint surfaces. This pain is due to irritation of the medial branch of the dorsal primary ramus, which innervates the facet joints. This medial branch is the target point of interventional pain procedures (medial branch block and radiofrequency ablation or neurotomy) to relieve facet joint pain. All branches of the dorsal primary ramus (medial, lateral, and intermediate) innervate the various paraspinal and deep muscles of the vertebral column.[103]

In addition to facet joint disorders, degenerative disk disease and disk displacement of varying degrees (bulging, protruding, and herniated) are conditions frequently regarded as generators of LBP. The facet joints and outer layer of the disks, together with the ligaments that support them, are richly innervated with small pain-sensitive (nociceptive) nerve fibers. This anatomical arrangement, together with the surge of chemical mediators released from pain-sensitive nerve fibers that occur during degeneration of the disk and facet joints or after an injury, explains why LBP can become disabling and protracted.

Neural innervations of the lumbar spine are derived from the sympathetic nervous system[Online2] and the somatic nervous system.[32,46,79,86,98,119] The sympathetic nerves are the sinuvertebral nerves (SVN), which, in addition to efferent fibers, provide nociceptive sensory fibers to the outer layer of the intervertebral disk, the ventral surface of the dura matter, periosteum of the spinal canal, and the posterior longitudinal ligaments.[Book1,2,6] The nucleus pulposus has no neural innervations. The SVN arose bilaterally and segmentally from the gray ramus communicans, and the fine sensory spinal branch arose from the ventral ramus. The conjoined nerves re-enter the intervertebral foramen and innervate the above structures, including the vertebral end plates and the segmental blood vessels (neurovascular plexus). The branches to the vertebral end plates become the basivertebral nerves, which in recent years have been the target point in the treatment of vertebrogenic pain using the radiofrequency ablation technique called "Intracept."[Online28-30] Most investigators have demonstrated that the SVN have up to three segmental levels of overlap, which explains why LBP is often diffuse and poorly localized. In view of the sympathetic nerve components of the SVN that innervate the lower lumbar disks via the L2 spinal nerve root, discogenic back pain is considered a form of "visceral" pain, a type of pain different from all other musculoskeletal pain. The initiation and transmission of pain are induced by ischemia, pressure, or inflammatory irritation. Psychological stress, which is so common among LBP sufferers, can activate the descending sympathetic nerve and lower their pain thresholds. Such a scenario may lead some healthcare providers to conclude that some LBP sufferers have concurrent psychological issues that complicate or augment their pain, which leads them to think of the old saying, "The pain is all in your head." However, it is an unfair characterization of patients with LBP, and given the physiological and anatomical association with the sympathetic nervous system, it is easy to understand the miseries of LBP sufferers.

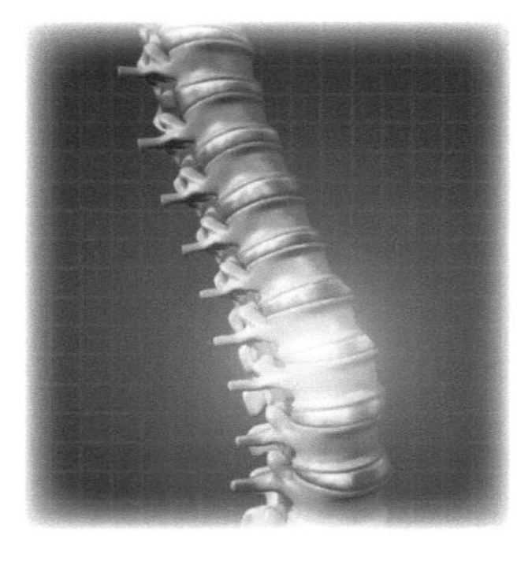

Unlike the cervical and thoracic segments of the spinal cord, which receive vascular supply from the single anterior spinal artery (which originates from the vertebral arteries) and two posterior spinal arteries, each segment of the upper four lumbar vertebrae receives blood supply from a pair of lumbar arteries that arise from the aorta. The fifth lumbar artery arises from the median sacral artery, which originates from the posterior branch of the distal segment of the abdominal aorta. The branches of these arteries supply the paravertebral muscles, and they form anastomoses around the facet joints and the spinous processes and laminae of the lumbar vertebrae.[Online1]

Intervertebral Disc

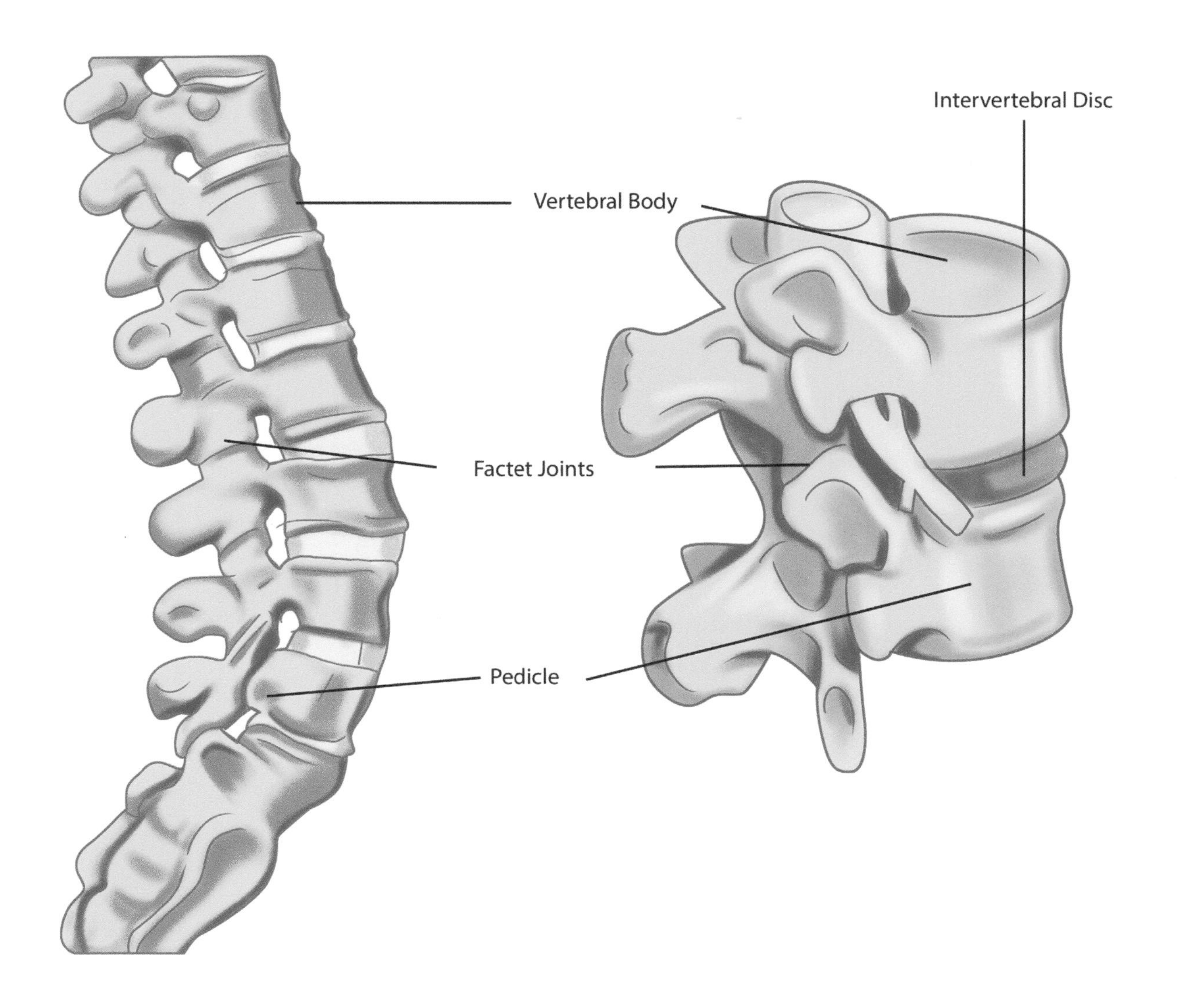

Sinuvertebral Nerve

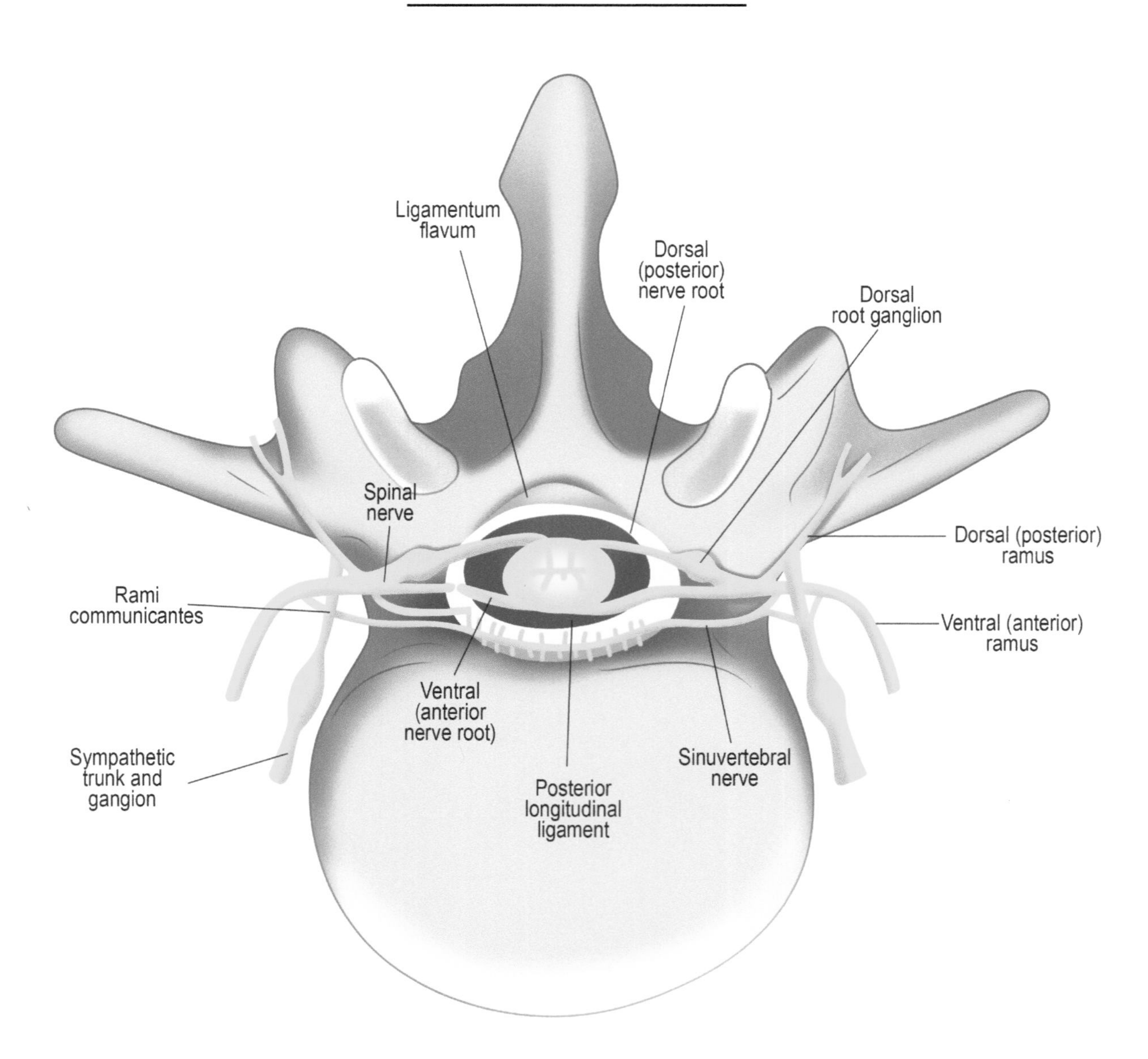

Blood supply of the lumbar spine

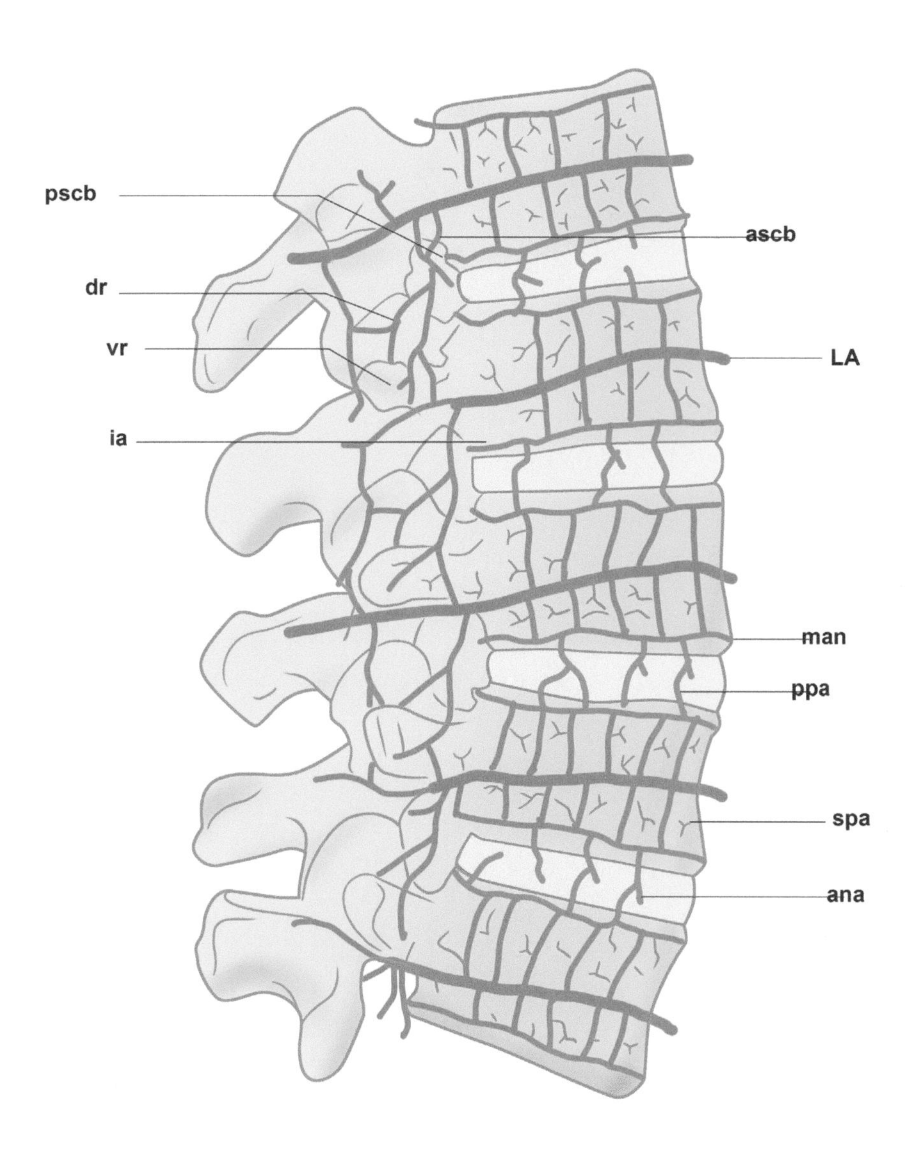

Sensory dermatomes of the lower extremities

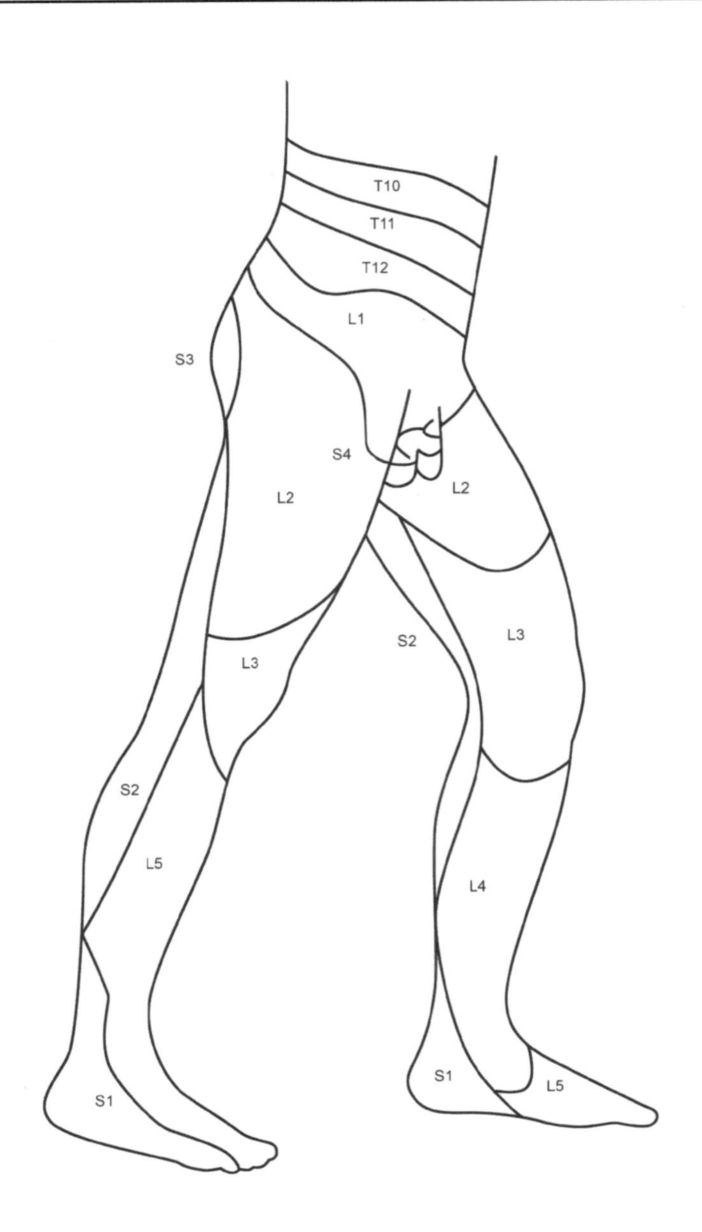

Lumbar Disc

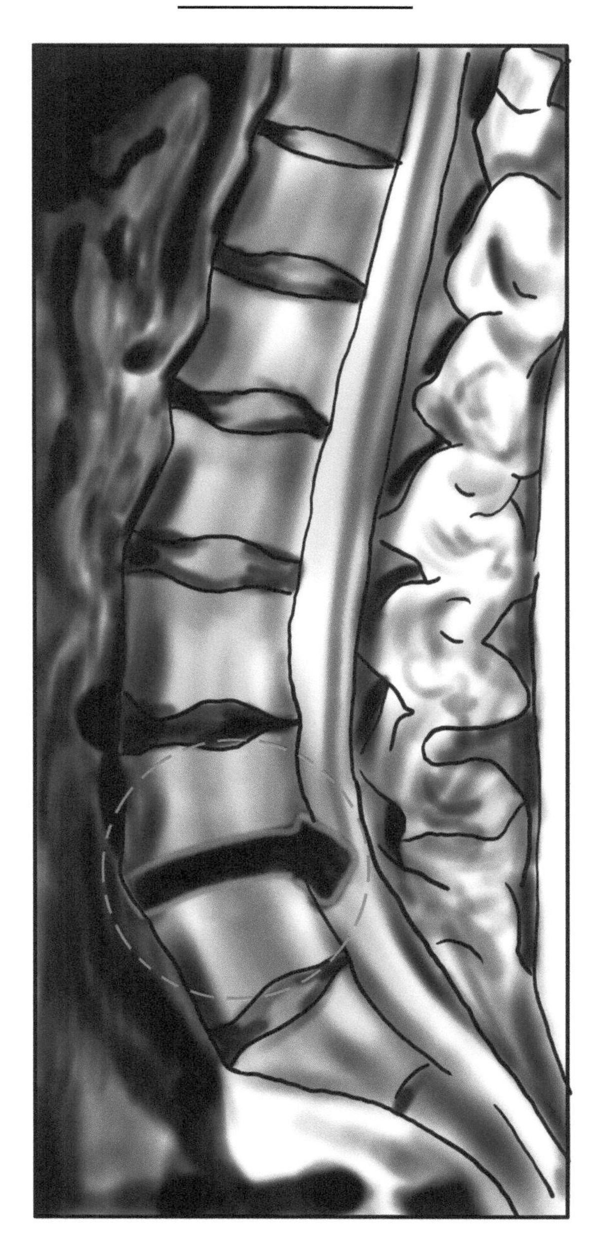

CHAPTER 3

Signs and symptoms of primary lumbar spine pathology and nerve root impingement

Please listen to the patient, he's trying to tell you what disease he has.

—Michael H. Brooke, M.D. (1934–2018), Professor of Neurology and Director, Jerry Lewis Neuromuscular Research Center, Washington University School of Medicine, St. Louis, Missouri

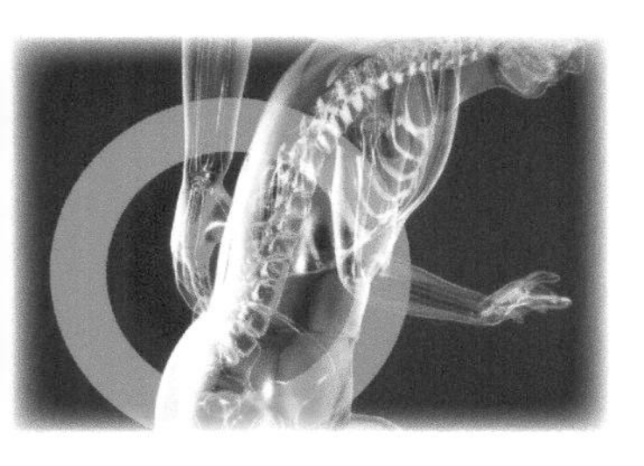

In general, the art of history-taking and the technique of clinical examination cannot be bypassed or replaced by the use of diagnostic procedures, which will always remain the bedrock of medical diagnosis. This is particularly true in the practice of neurology, where each symptom represents a manifestation of an impairment or malfunction of a certain component(s) of either (or both) the central or peripheral nervous system. Therefore, good knowledge of the anatomy and physiology of the nervous system is the key to asking pertinent questions during the process of history-taking. It can be a disconcerting situation when a clinician is not making eye contact with the patient and is busy staring at the medical chart or laptop computer while the patient is struggling to relay his or her history in detail while feeling quite uncomfortable and miserable on the examining table because of LBP. The ramifications are obvious. There are, of course, certain straightforward conditions when the history is clearly diagnostic and the laboratory findings are confirmatory. Regardless, the need to put together the clinical findings and the results of laboratory test procedures that are vital in the formulation of the treatment plan cannot be overstated.

Identification of the generator of LBP is not easy because there are no specific diagnostic features of certain vertebral disease processes. Radiologic signs of degenerative disk disease can be seen in the general population, especially in the elderly, and mild degeneration can be seen in people in their teens. Likewise, varying degrees of disk displacement can be asymptomatic or, if present, do not necessarily imply causality. Regardless, disk degeneration and displacement can induce mechanical or axial pain with or without signs of nerve root impingement.[22,24,27,39,78,80,87] Axial pain is described as pain that aggravates during sitting, standing, and bending and recedes partially during recumbency.

Facet joint disorders are characterized by dull localized LBP that may extend to the buttocks, hips, knees, or thighs without sensory loss or changes in the muscle stretch reflexes.[52,96] Local tenderness can be elicited in the lower back. The pain is usually more pronounced during the early morning hours or after strenuous exercises. Prolonged driving can exacerbate pain. Bending may sometimes partially relieve the pain. Engaging in poor posture, vehicular accidents, and sports-related injuries are common precipitating factors.

Bone spurs or osteophytes, considered a reaction to chronic mechanical stress, are common radiological findings, and can be asymptomatic. At some point, they may become symptomatic when the spinal canal becomes narrow (stenosis), impinges on a spinal nerve, or directly irritates the muscles and tendons.[57] When the neural foramen becomes significantly narrowed, compression of a nerve root can lead to various symptoms stemming from the impairment of sensory and motor fibers. When the spinal canal is severely narrowed, a condition known as "neurogenic claudication," or pseudoclaudication, develops. This condition is characterized by leg pain that occurs when walking. It can mimic vascular claudication, a condition that is common among patients with circulatory disturbances, particularly atherosclerosis.

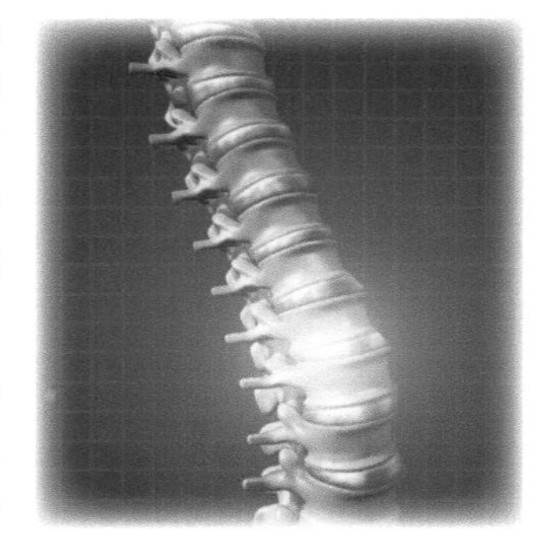

Besides disk degeneration, facet joint disorders, osteoporosis, and osteophyte formation, another degenerative process that can cause LBP is spondylolisthesis, which is the anterior or forward displacement of one vertebra relative to another or the vertebra (or sacrum) below it. It occurs at the L5 vertebra in the majority of cases. Such a situation can generate LBP because of the deformity and narrowing of the vertebral canal. This condition is likely to occur following a stress fracture in the vertebra, also known as spondylolysis. Young people who participate in sports are at risk of developing spondylolysis and spondylolisthesis. Age (after age 50) and genetics are other risk factors. Leg and buttock pain and bladder disturbances are common symptoms.[41]

One particular spinal deformity that is frequently encountered in the field of neuromuscular disorders is scoliosis. This condition is a frequent and unavoidable consequence of muscle weakness seen in congenital neuromuscular disorders such as congenital muscular dystrophy,[62] congenital fiber type disproportion, nemaline myopathy, central core disease, myotubular myopathy, and spinal muscular atrophy.[Book7,8] Unlike the scoliosis encountered in patients without neuromuscular disorders, the treatment approach must be individualized because of the risk of complications with some type of anesthetics. One particular type of congenital muscle disorder at risk for malignant hyperthermia is central core disease. However, patients who are being considered for possible surgery for some type of spine pathology but with unexplained and persistently elevated creatine kinase muscle enzyme must be screened and tested for the risk of malignant hyperthermia.[111] All anesthesiologists are very much aware of this life-threatening condition that results from exposure to volatile anesthetic agents and depolarizing muscle relaxants. It is characterized by tachycardia, tachypnea, hyperthermia, hypercapnia, acidosis, muscle rigidity, and rhabdomyolysis (severe muscle breakdown). Kidney failure can result from rhabdomyolysis and myoglobinuria.

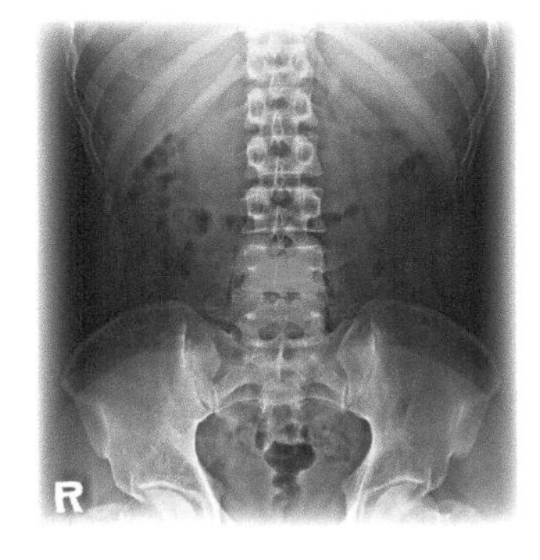

A systemic rheumatologic disorder whose etiology remains unknown is ankylosing spondylitis (AS). The word is derived from Greek *ankylos*, meaning crooked, and *spondylos*, meaning vertebra. It has other names that include Marie-Strumpell arthritis, Bechterew's disease, and Pierre-Marie's disease. It is characterized by inflammation of joints in the entire spine and ossification of the outer fibers of the intervertebral disks, which gives the spine a bamboo appearance in x-rays as the disease progresses. Diffuse back pain and stiffness of the affected joints (shoulders, hips, knees, and sacroiliacs) worsen over time. AS begins insidiously in young adults without sex predilection. Some patients develop eye symptoms (anterior uveitis) along with cardiopulmonary involvement, the latter being the most common cause of death. It is prevalent in northern European countries. There is no cure for this disease. Various anti-inflammatory drugs and physical therapy are the mainstays of symptomatic therapy. Severe cases may require surgery using knee or hip joint replacements. In recent years, monoclonal antibodies have been used with encouraging results.[9] One particular monoclonal antibody, secukinumab, has been approved for the treatment of AS by the Food and Drug Administration (FDA) and the European Union.[Online17]

The generators of LBP, as discussed above, are only one aspect of lumbar spine disorders. When one or more spinal nerves are affected by a degenerative process or injury, the diagnosis and treatment approach, including prognosis, may change because the treating healthcare professional has to deal with both the mechanical issue (axial pain) and the spinal nerve(s) affected. Basically, a nerve bundle has motor, sensory, and autonomic fiber components. A peripheral nerve bundle is actually derived from the merging of various nerve roots. To make it riveting, a lesion affecting a nerve root will give rise to signs and symptoms different from a lesion that affects a peripheral nerve trunk. Regardless of whether the site of lesion is in the nerve root (medically termed "radiculopathy") or peripheral nerve (medically termed "peripheral neuropathy"), those nerve fibers within the bundle—motor, sensory, and autonomic—will malfunction. Therefore, the clinical abnormalities will reflect the impairment to the function of those nerve fibers, and they consist of weakness (motor fibers), tingling and numbness (sensory fibers), and a cold or warm sensation with or without changes in the local sweating pattern (autonomic fibers)—all of which may occur in various degrees and proportions.

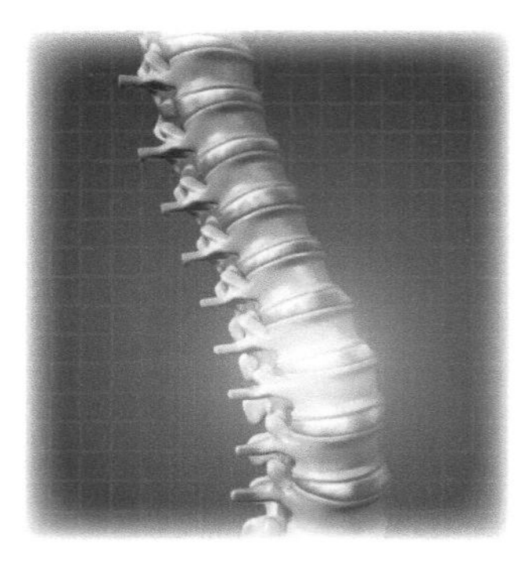

The pattern of sensory loss or deficit in nerve root impingement is characteristic and is felt in a band-like distribution on the skin (dermatome) of the thigh, leg, and foot (anterior aspect of the thigh in L2–3; anterolateral aspect of the thigh, medial surface of the leg and inner aspect of the big toe in L4; lateral aspect of the thigh and leg and top of the foot and the middle toes in L5; and posterior aspect of the thigh and leg and lateral surface of the foot and small toe in S1). Depending on the severity of impingement, the focal muscle weakness is either felt by the patient or detected by the examiner (weakness of the anterior muscle of the thigh in L3 or L4, weakness of the hamstring, ankle, or big toe dorsiflexor in L5, and weakness of the plantar flexor in S1). Drooping of the big toe in association with LBP, even if the sensory deficit is not well defined, is a diagnostic marker for L5 radiculopathy.[73] Another neurologic deficit that identifies the nerve root affected is a change in the muscle stretch reflex—absent or depressed in the patella and ankle in L3–4 and S1 radiculopathies, respectively. In L5, changes in the reflex may not be evident, except for the hamstring reflex, which can be difficult to elicit or gauge.

One must be cognizant of the fact that HD and LBP are two different clinical and pathologic entities, but they can be mutually inclusive in most cases of spine injury because the mechanical stress exerted on the spine through trauma will likely irritate the SVN in the spine, the neural innervations of the facet joints, the ligaments, and the myofascial compartment surrounding the spine. When the intervertebral disk is displaced significantly, the spinal nerve is liable to be compressed and compromise the various nerve fibers within the nerve trunk. The occurrence of disk herniation with radiculopathy but without LBP can be explained by the location of the herniation—the spinal nerve root being compressed is proximal to the branching point of the SVN and the afferent pathways for the discogenic LBP are not in the spinal nerve at the same level.

One particular and intriguing constellation of symptoms that is not well recognized and is frequently overlooked in LBP consists of cold and swollen sensations in the lower extremities, at times associated with reddish discoloration of the skin. These symptoms are mediated by the sympathetic nerve fibers, and are termed vasomotor symptoms. They are experienced by some patients with axial LBP, particularly stemming from discopathies, are either unilateral or bilateral, are steady or intermittent, and are without dermatomal distribution. Such phenomenology is not well recognized but is worthy of diagnostic consideration. Why is that so? The SVN is actually a sympathetic nerve that mediates vasomotor symptoms, so it is not surprising that these symptoms are likely to develop in disk disease.

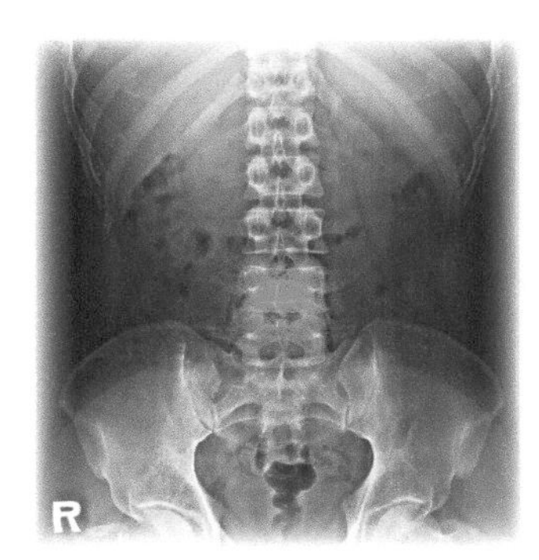

In this era of space exploration, healthcare professionals specializing in the spine know full well that the biomechanics and anatomy of the spine are altered among astronauts during space flights.[93] Pain can occur when the spine lengthens in microgravity. The resulting pain stems from stress on the disks and various vertebral articulations innervated by the sinuvertebral nerves and nociceptive nerve fibers that originate from the dorsal root ganglia. This stress is the result of the supraphysiologic swelling of the intervertebral disks due to the removal of gravitational compressive loads in microgravity. Upon landing, the spine re-adapts to gravity and reverts back to its original length. [Online18] Some astronauts may continue to experience LBP, while others do not. During a protracted stay in the international space station or a trip to Mars lasting several months, astronauts have to deal with other medical conditions besides the spine—some serious and life threatening—such as cardiac arrhythmia, heart attack, stroke, leg thrombosis and pulmonary embolism, appendicitis, and various gastrointestinal disorders that can present acutely, as well as systemic infections.

CHAPTER 4

Diseases and other conditions that can cause or are associated with low back pain

> Strength does not come from winning. Your struggles develop when you go through hardships and decide not to surrender. That is strength.
>
> *—Arnold Schwarzenegger, actor, former politician, and bodybuilder*

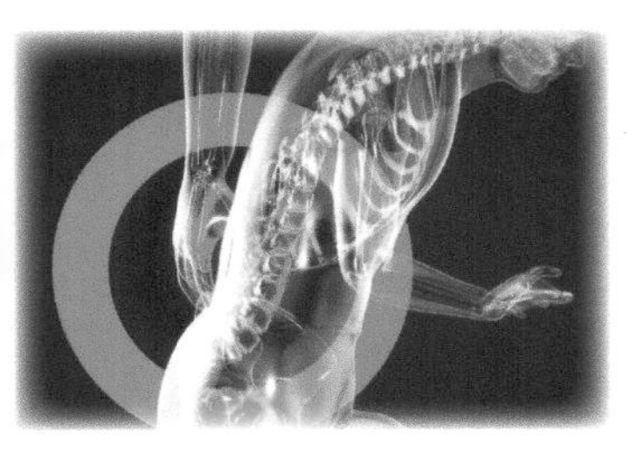

All things considered, the clinical and laboratory findings in LBP sufferers can be easily correlated with each other, and appropriate therapy instituted accordingly. However, the success (or failure) of certain treatment modalities is a separate issue that may vary from clinic to clinic or hospital to hospital. In some situations, the correlation may not be straightforward, to say the least. In this situation, it behooves the healthcare provider to search for clear causative factors related to LBP in order for treatment to succeed. Other than the well-known primary spinal disorders that can cause LBP, other conditions, if left undiagnosed, particularly those related to malignancy or meningeal carcinomatosis, can be problematic and precarious. As alluded to in the foregoing discussion, the art of history-taking and meticulous clinical examination are the key to a correct diagnosis and/or the success of a treatment modality.

More often than not, someone complaining of LBP is likely to be diagnosed with disk disease, osteoarthritis, and various degenerative bone disorders. However, conditions exist that may present with atypical symptomatology. If the symptoms are not attributed to injuries or occupational factors, tend to exacerbate regardless of body position but, especially during nocturnal hours, are accompanied by focal sensory and motor weakness, including bladder disturbances, and remain persistent despite extensive therapy, further diagnostic evaluation is in order. In this situation, imaging with either a CAT scan or MRI may reveal a neoplastic process, particularly a primary spinal tumor, which may be located in the vertebra, meninges, nerve root, or parenchyma of the spinal cord. Since the spinal cord ends at L1, an intraparenchymal (intramedullary) tumor is expected to occur in the thoracic and cervical cord. In the lumbar spine, the tumor can be located in the meninges (intradural-extramedullary), between the meninges and vertebra (extradural), or within the substance of the vertebra. Spinal tumors are either benign or malignant. Spinal tumors that are extradural are usually metastatic, and less commonly benign schwannomas. The bony spinal column is the most common site of metastasis from cancer of the lungs and breast, followed by multiple myeloma, melanoma, and sarcoma. The most common primary tumor within the vertebra is hemangioma, which rarely produces pain.

In many cases, a history of an injury provides a good clue to the cause of LBP, but in its absence, along with the presence of systemic signs like fever and general body malaise, an infectious process clearly comes to the mind of an astute examiner. If diagnosed early, an infectious process such as osteomyelitis can be treated appropriately with antibiotics and surgery in some cases. Epidural abscesses may present with weakness, sensory loss, and impaired bladder control. Those at risk for developing epidural abscesses are diabetics, people who are immune compromised, drug addicts, alcoholics, and post-lumbar surgery patients. If treated appropriately, the deficits can be reversed or minimized.

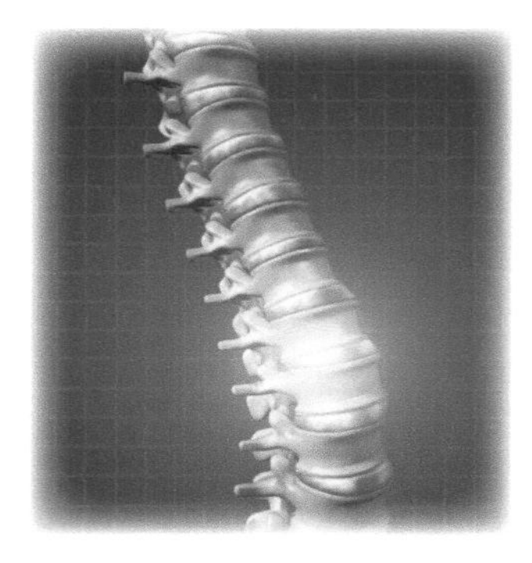

Spinal cord infarction can present with back pain accompanied by paralysis and sensory loss in the upper and lower extremities, depending on the level of infarction. It can be caused by aortic disease (dissection and aneurysm), vertebral artery dissection, embolism, trauma, hypercoagulable state, arteriovenous malformation, vasculitis, and abscess.

Lyme disease, a tick-borne illness transmitted to mammals through the bite of an infected tick vector (Ixodes scapularis), can affect both the central and peripheral nervous systems, and back pain can be a presenting symptom. LBP can occur when the spirochete bacteria (Borrelia burgdorferi) invade multiple spinal nerve roots, including cranial nerves. On rare occasions, isolated weakness of the lower extremity, owing to involvement of the femoral nerve, can cause gait difficulty.[66] Timely diagnosis and treatment with antibiotics can minimize or reverse the damage caused by bacteria.

Multi-nerve root involvement (termed polyradiculopathy), a clinicopathologic hallmark of Guillain–Barre syndrome, and an acute or subacute autoimmune peripheral nerve disorder that affects myelin (outer coating of peripheral nerves and nerve roots) can present with back pain. The clinical symptomatology and examination findings are easily recognizable. Laboratory diagnosis is achieved by a spinal fluid examination and a peripheral nerve conduction examination. The hallmarks of this condition include high protein content in the spinal fluid with very little cellular presence, along with very slowed peripheral nerves (or nerve root conduction via F-waves) due to the impairment of saltatory conduction.

Multiple sclerosis, an autoimmune central nervous system disorder that affects the myelin coating of the nerve fiber tracts, can produce back pain. The exact mechanism is uncertain, but muscle spasticity and resulting mechanical stress on the musculoskeletal system are significant factors. Theoretically, the presence of a demyelinating plaque in proximity to the entry of the dorsal root may induce back pain.

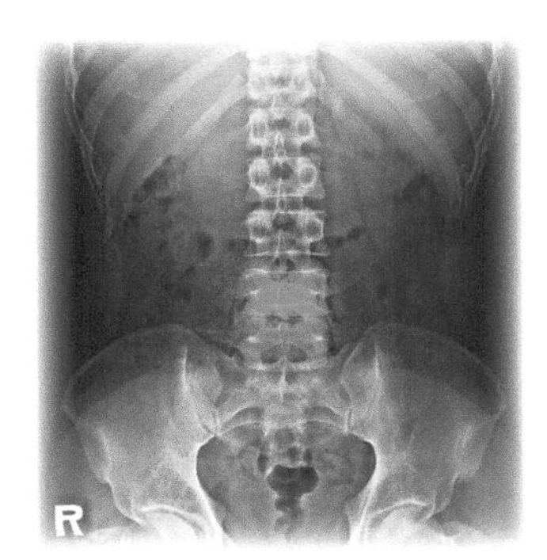

Referred pain from renal stones, urinary bladder and prostate infection, and endometriosis are extra-spinal conditions that can be easily diagnosed clinically through radiographic procedures and blood work.

Owing to changes in the biomechanics of the lumbar spine and pelvis during pregnancy, LBP is not uncommon. Physiologic causes include a shift in the center of gravity, an increase in hormone levels, and weight gain. Physical therapy, correction of poor posture, heat, ice, and massage, and flexing the knees when supine or lying on either side can minimize LBP.

Fibromyalgia (FM), a common rheumatologic disorder, can present with back pain. This condition is characterized by multiple and generalized musculoskeletal pain associated with sleep disturbances, chronic fatigue, memory problems, and difficulty concentrating. In some cases, this condition has an underlying involvement of small-diameter nerve fibers, also known as small-fiber neuropathy (SFN), a neurologic condition that affects nerve fibers that mediate pain sensation and autonomic function.[81, Online23-26] SFN has diverse etiologies that include diabetes, autoimmune diseases, metabolic and endocrine diseases, particularly hypothyroidism, coronavirus infection, connective tissue diseases, cancer, amyloid sensory neuropathy, and Fabry's disease (a genetic lysosomal disease that affects several parts of the body, including the skin, heart, and kidneys). The presence of SFN explains why some people with FM may complain of local tenderness in the skin and underlying muscles and fibrous tissues, including the lower back. Proper identification of this condition can avoid the use of unnecessary and inappropriate test procedures for LBP.

In summary, symptoms that constitute "red flags" should alert all healthcare providers when dealing with patients with back pain, even in the presence of primary vertebral pathology. These symptoms include severe nocturnal back pain, chronic weight loss, fever, urogenital disturbances, and diffuse lower extremity weakness. In other situations, LBP can sometimes mask the signs and symptoms of a central nervous system disorder, but a good neurological examination can circumvent misdiagnosis and ensure that appropriate diagnostic procedures are administered.

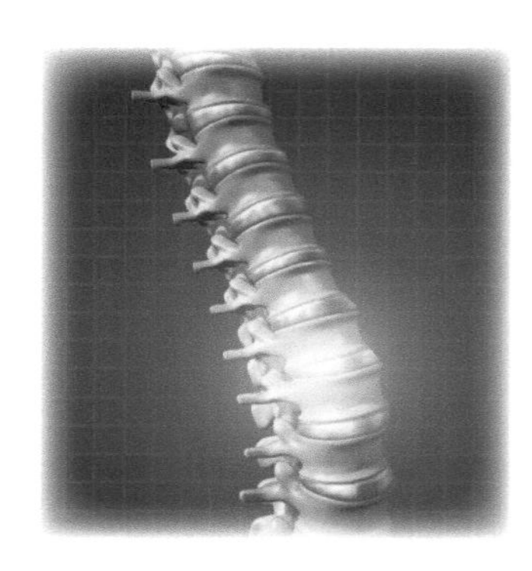

CHAPTER 5

Diagnostic tests and the consequences of misdiagnoses and misapplications—Helpful and Unhelpful Laboratory Procedures

The best way of handling pain is to study it objectively.

—Arthur C. Clarke (1917–2008), British Science writer, inventor, futurits

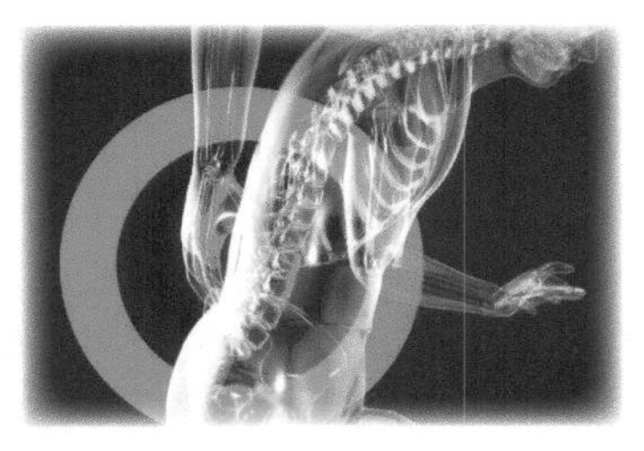

In the past, the diagnosis and management of LBP were based on the results of clinical examination and plain x-rays. If necessary, LBP sufferers were subjected to an invasive procedure called myelography, a procedure that involves lumbar puncture to instill intrathecal contrast agent to outline the spinal canal and nerve roots, and to look for HD. Some patients were referred to the electromyography (EMG) clinic to diagnose or identify the affected nerve root. The technique of myelography has evolved in subsequent years with the use of less toxic contrast material, but in recent years, its use in the routine evaluation of spinal disease has been replaced by either a CAT scan or MRI. Nevertheless, it remains a valuable procedure in select cases (especially when combined with a CAT scan), such as arachnoid diseases (cyst and inflammation), metastatic cancer, spinal stenosis, nerve root avulsion, and spinal fluid leak.[100,113]

CAT scan and MRI are equally valuable; the former utilizes radiation that is considered safe for adults, while the latter uses a harmless magnetic field and pulses of radio waves, and both are painless. There is a theoretical risk to the fetus during the first trimester for both procedures. For those who are claustrophobic, do not respond to sedatives, and have cardiac pacemakers and other metal implants, CAT scan is an alternative option. CAT scan is more effective in demonstrating bone pathology (arthritis and fractures), calcified soft tissues, and blood vessels. MRI is useful in detecting abnormalities in the disk anatomy, spinal cord, and soft tissue organs. In recent years, an upright MRI technique has been devised to detect disk displacement, which is not evident in a conventional supine MRI. According to most radiologists, the technique can bring the symptoms on when a patient is in an upright position, symptoms that are not present (or less intense) in a recumbent position. When viewed in upright MRI, the reproduction of the symptoms correlates with the disk displacement that has become more evident compared to conventional techniques.[Online19] Apparently, the pressure exerted on the already compromised posterior longitudinal ligaments increases during an upright position, making borderline disk displacement (or bulging disk) appear more distinct or herniated. A case history is presented below.

A sixty-two-year-old man was involved in a two-car accident and developed diffuse pain from the cervical down to the lumbar spine. There was no prior history of spinal injury, LBP, or neck pain, and his medical history was essentially unremarkable. Plain x-rays of his entire spine showed straightening of the cervical lordosis and several desiccated disks and osteoarthritis in the lumbar spine (L3–4 and L4–5). His cervical pain improved with the intake of oral analgesics, physical therapy, and massage, but he continued to complain of non-radicular LBP that tended to intensify when standing or walking. A conventional MRI of the lumbar spine showed mild bulging disks, as previously demonstrated in the CAT scan, together with desiccated disks at the same level, and bulging disks at T6–7 and T9–10. He later underwent an upright MRI that showed multiple HDs at the abovementioned levels. He declined to undergo a surgical evaluation. Two months later, his insurance company sent him to an independent medical examiner (IME), who wrote a report stating that the x-rays and MRI findings were consistent with the aging process and that he did not sustain any injuries related to the accident. Therefore, no further evaluation or therapy were necessary. Unfortunately, for some unclear reason, the IME did not mention or make any comments on the findings demonstrated in the upright spine MRI imaging, which showed multiple HDs. The injured sought legal help, and after a year of suffering from persistent pain despite multiple interventional treatments, his case was presented to the local court. The jury ruled in his favor after the expert witness presented medical evidence that supported his claim. He prevailed in the Court of Law. He continued to receive conservative therapy for his chronic pain years after the court settlement.

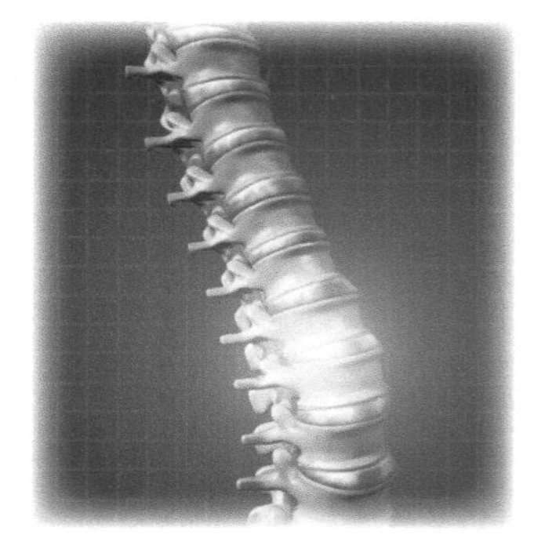

Both CAT scans and MRI usually require an injection of contrast materials to improve tissue contrast and visualization of the pathology being studied. These contrast materials may induce allergic and systemic reactions along with renal complications related to gadolinium, which is used for MRI scanning.[Online12] Gadolinium, which can accumulate in tissues and organs such as the bone, brain, and liver, can be neurotoxic, especially when administered to patients with neurological disorders secondary to elevated or toxic levels of zinc. A rare case of pancreatitis has been reported.

It is noteworthy that there are asymptomatic cases of disk degeneration and/or disk displacement.[55] Conversely, LBP can occur with minimal disk changes. As discussed in the previous chapters, other structures in the spine can generate pain when irritated or inflamed. In one recent observational study, the presence of sympathetically mediated symptoms (cold and warm sensations, intermittent swelling, and reddish discoloration in the lower extremities) may point to a pathologic disk as the source of LBP. This is unsurprising, given that the sympathetic nerves (SVN) innervate the intervertebral disks.[94] If this clinical observation is further confirmed, the presence of such symptoms may provide a strong clinical indication and justification to perform lumbar discograms for LBP sufferers who fail to improve with conservative measures.

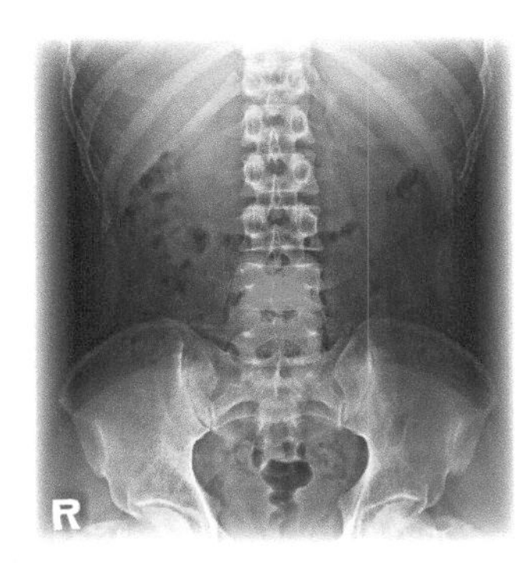

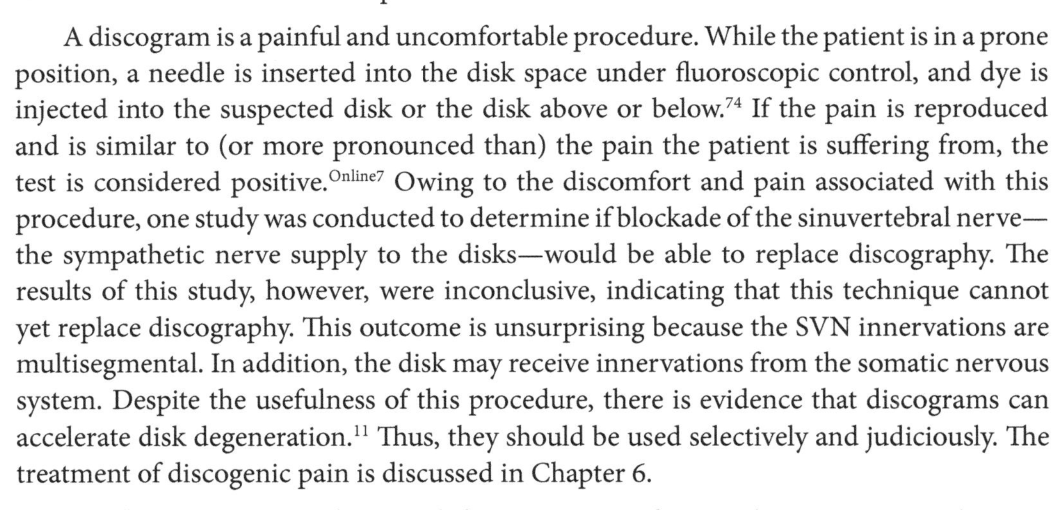

A discogram is a painful and uncomfortable procedure. While the patient is in a prone position, a needle is inserted into the disk space under fluoroscopic control, and dye is injected into the suspected disk or the disk above or below.[74] If the pain is reproduced and is similar to (or more pronounced than) the pain the patient is suffering from, the test is considered positive.[Online7] Owing to the discomfort and pain associated with this procedure, one study was conducted to determine if blockade of the sinuvertebral nerve—the sympathetic nerve supply to the disks—would be able to replace discography. The results of this study, however, were inconclusive, indicating that this technique cannot yet replace discography. This outcome is unsurprising because the SVN innervations are multisegmental. In addition, the disk may receive innervations from the somatic nervous system. Despite the usefulness of this procedure, there is evidence that discograms can accelerate disk degeneration.[11] Thus, they should be used selectively and judiciously. The treatment of discogenic pain is discussed in Chapter 6.

Another diagnostic tool to search for a generator of LBP is the SPECT scan. This scan is a sensitive test that can detect facet joint disorders, stress fractures in the spine, and disk infections. It is an expensive test procedure, consisting of the injection of a radionuclide, which accumulates in the body part suspected to be the source of pain or abnormal metabolism. The body is then scanned for gamma rays being emitted from inflamed tissues, and the images are displayed in color. Although the amount of radioactive material is minimal, the procedure must be avoided in pregnant women. The radioactive tracer is eliminated from the body within two days, but the elimination can be facilitated by increasing fluid intake.

Clinically, insofar as vasomotor symptoms are concerned, it should be noted that facet joints, which are innervated by the nociceptive fibers from the dorsal root ganglia, also receive innervations from the paravertebral sympathetic nerve ganglia. Therefore, when a patient reports these symptoms in the setting of back pain, facet joint irritation must also be considered in the differential diagnosis. In animal studies, innervations of the joints from the paraverterbral sympathetic ganglia have been demonstrated in rats using the retrograde neural tracer transport method.

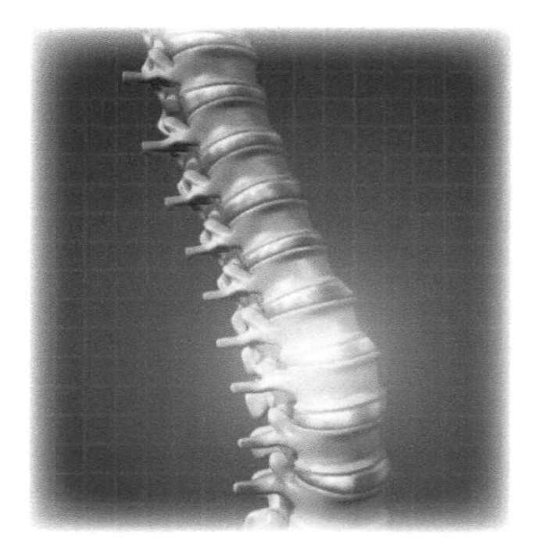

Physiologically, pain stemming from any part of the body, particularly the soft tissues, muscles, and bones in the spine, is associated with vasomotor changes emanating from the affected area. The area is either warm or cold, and these temperature changes can be detected using liquid crystal thermographs or digital infrared thermal imaging. The discovery of thermal radiation is a significant milestone in the diagnosis and treatment of various disorders, such as LBP, headache, breast disease, dental conditions, peripheral nerve injuries, vascular diseases, carotid artery disease, and complex regional pain syndrome. This thermal radiation was discovered by William Herschel, a musician and astronomer who discovered the planet Uranus. While investigating the problems of optical glass design for his astronomy project, he set up an experiment to determine the heating effects on the eye. To project a visible spectrum, he used a prism set on a blacked-out window and placed thermometers in each of the color bands. After repeating the experiments several times, he established a consistent rise in temperature beyond the visible red end of the spectrum. He called it "dark heat" or infrared radiation. This is the basis for the use of thermal imaging or infrared thermographs using thermal cameras.

In recent years, thermal imaging has not been well received as a diagnostic procedure, and several test procedures have superseded it, but is totally painless. [Online13-16] It can be expensive, depending on the extent of the procedure, and few health insurance companies cover the expense. This procedure is beset with controversies, bureaucracies, and politics; however, it provides incontrovertible evidence for the existence of body reactions to pain and is, therefore, useful in distinguishing true pain from malingering pain. In LBP associated with radicular symptoms, thermal imaging can demonstrate the "dermatomal" (thermographers use the term "thermatome") distribution of sensory deficits. However, this aspect of thermal imaging used in various pain syndromes can generate controversies in the legal system, particularly in vehicular accidents and workers' compensation cases. The procedure has been vilified because of reported abuse and misuse by some healthcare practitioners.

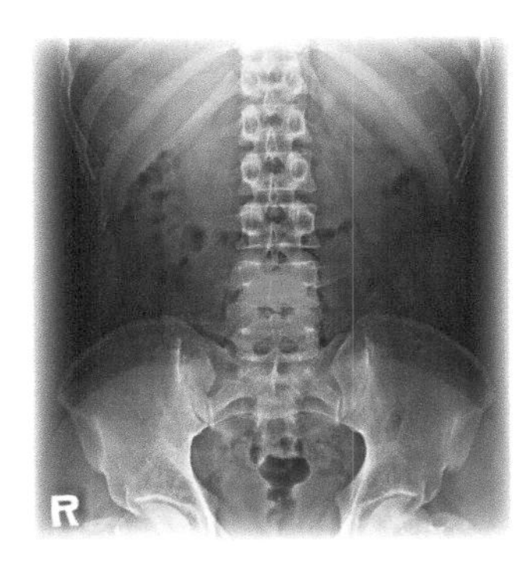

A physiologic test procedure that is very frequently performed in LBP is an EMG and peripheral nerve conduction examination. This test procedure is performed by various medical specialties, including neurologists, physiatrists, physical therapists, and some chiropractors. EMG, as the name indicates, is a recording of motor unit activity, particularly the muscle fibers innervated by the motor axon. It is a well-established diagnostic procedure that is useful in the diagnosis of various muscle and motor unit disorders. However, its utility in the diagnosis of pain per se and pain stemming from musculoskeletal disorders is questionable, to say the least, because EMG can only assess the motor axons and muscle fiber activities but not the sensory axis of the neuromuscular system. Moreover, pain generated from the facet joints, discopathies, irritation of the ligaments, tendons, bones, and myofascial tissues cannot be assessed by this method. Some investigators have elicited "abnormalities" in EMG patterns in myofascial pain, but these findings do not represent denervation, which is the hallmark of muscles deprived of nerve supply. Denervation is defined as the presence of fibrillation potentials and sharp positive waves. In chronic situations, complex motor units and high-frequency motor discharges are displayed on the EMG screen. Nevertheless, these so-called abnormalities elicited from myofascial tissues are simply manifestations of motor impairment resulting from irritable and painful muscles, and they do not directly reflect the activity of nociceptive nerve fibers (pain fibers). Another disconcerting and uncomfortable situation for patients is the aggressive approach by some electromyographers to sample the paraspinal muscles in search of abnormalities. It is unimaginable to insert a long EMG needle into painful and spastic lumbar muscles in a patient already complaining of severe LBP, along with realizing that this procedure does not and cannot assess pain directly. Moreover, even in the absence of anticoagulation, hematoma from needle insertion is not uncommon. Anecdotally, some patients develop complex regional pain following extensive needle insertion. Another disconcerting aspect of this procedure is the number of muscles tested, which can range from a minimum of four muscles to as many as twenty muscles in the extremities, depending on the training, education, and aggressiveness of the electromyographer. In conclusion, when the clinical examination findings are clearly and unequivocally diagnostic of radiculopathy, EMG is either optional or unnecessary. Moreover, when the muscle strength is normal, there is no sensory loss, and the muscle stretch reflexes are intact, there is a very good chance that the EMG will yield normal findings. A good neurological examination, therefore, should determine the need to order or perform this procedure. It does not stand alone as a diagnostic procedure.[63,64,67,69]

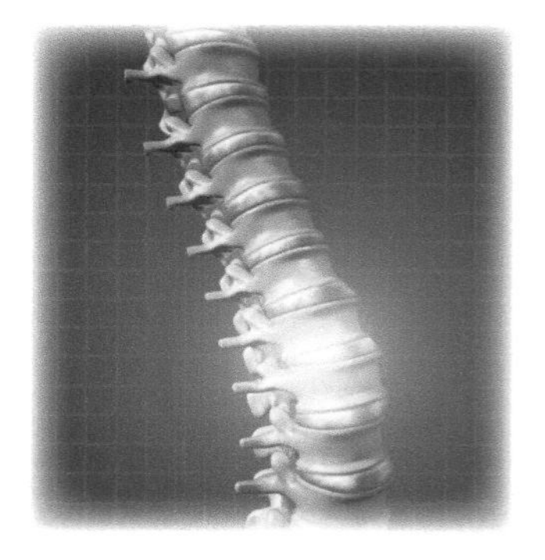

With regard to peripheral nerve conduction examination, this particular part of electrodiagnosis in suspected radiculopathy is practically useless. It is usually performed on a limited basis in routine evaluations, but an extensive nerve conduction examination in the absence of clinical signs or symptoms of peripheral neuropathy is unnecessary. Likewise, nerve conduction procedures to elicit "F-wave" and "H-reflex" responses are either useless or unnecessary when the clinical neurological examination findings are normal, or unless there are signs of proximal demyelinating polyneuropathy, a condition that can be diagnosed with a good clinical history and examination. An F-wave response is a low-amplitude late motor action potential originally elicited from the small muscles of the foot, although it can be elicited by supramaximal electrical stimulation of any motor or mixed nerve. It is a pure motor response that follows the compound muscle action potential. Thus, it is of no value to assess pain directly, not to mention that it is an uncomfortable part of peripheral electrodiagnosis because of the large amount of electrical current needed to elicit the response. The H-reflex (or Hoffmann's reflex) involves afferent and efferent loops. It is the analogue of the ankle reflex, which is mediated by the S1 root and elicited by tapping the Achilles tendon. Therefore, if the ankle reflex is absent or hypoactive and the gastrocnemius muscle is weak or denervated, electrical elicitation of the H-reflex is unnecessary.

Another less helpful procedure in LBP syndromes is somatosensory evoked responses (SEPs). This procedure involves electrical stimulation of the peroneal and tibial nerves in the lower extremity, and the median and ulnar nerves in the upper extremity. The average of multiple responses is recorded over the contralateral scalp. It should be noted that this procedure is of no value in pain syndromes because it can only assess the integrity of large-diameter fibers, nerve fibers that do not carry or transmit pain impulses. It is tedious and time consuming. Therefore, unless large fibers are involved, this procedure will yield normal findings. Many practitioners, including me, abandoned doing this procedure many years ago. However, if there is a question of intraparenchymal nerve fiber tract pathology in the spinal cord, such as in multiple sclerosis, neoplasm, or transverse myelopathy, this procedure can be informative. Again, a good clinical examination is crucial to justify its use.

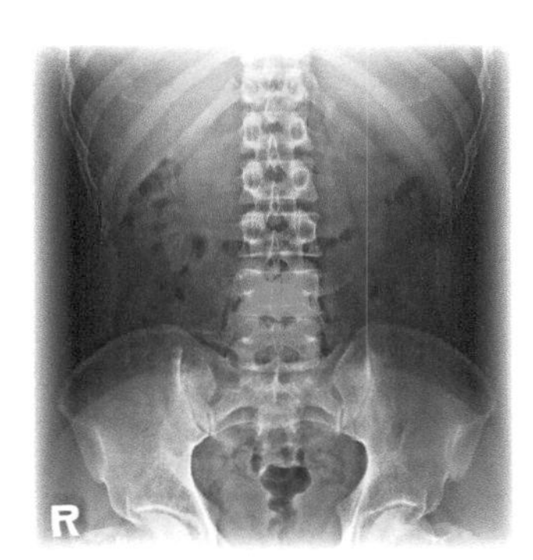

Legally, in pursuit of objective findings that correlate with the history and examination findings in an injured patient, especially in those with non-diagnostic and non-conclusive laboratory test findings, some practitioners may be pressured as a last resort to order some test procedures to look for "abnormalities" that may be causally related to the injury. Although such practices can be considered patient-oriented, they can be interpreted differently by some healthcare practitioners. A case history is presented below.

A 50-year-old right-handed man, a construction worker, developed LBP while lifting a heavy load. The pain was severe, forcing him to go to a local emergency room. It extended to the right leg and foot. He was diagnosed with acute lumbar strain. His medical history was otherwise unremarkable. Subsequent laboratory investigations revealed normal lumbar spine x-rays and two bulging disks in MRI. The LBP persisted despite rest, intake of oral analgesics, and physical therapy. He was later advised to return to work with physical limitations. However, his employer terminated his job because he was required only if he could work at full capacity. He consulted a chiropractor and was put on total disability. He later underwent thermal imaging of the lumbar spine, which showed a hot spot in the lower back and focal hypothermia in the distribution of the L4 dermatome. These findings were submitted as evidence to the Workers' Compensation Board, indicating that he had nerve root irritation and musculoskeletal injury to explain his job-related symptoms. However, the evidence was disallowed because thermal imaging was declared an invalid test procedure.

CHAPTER 6

Conservative and interventional treatments—What is the natural history of an untreated herniated lumbar disk?

There is a saying in Tibetan, tragedy should be utilized as a source of strength. No matter what sort of difficulties, how painful the experience is, we lose our hope, that's our real disaster.

—Dalai Lama

There are no gains without pains.

—Benjamin Franklin

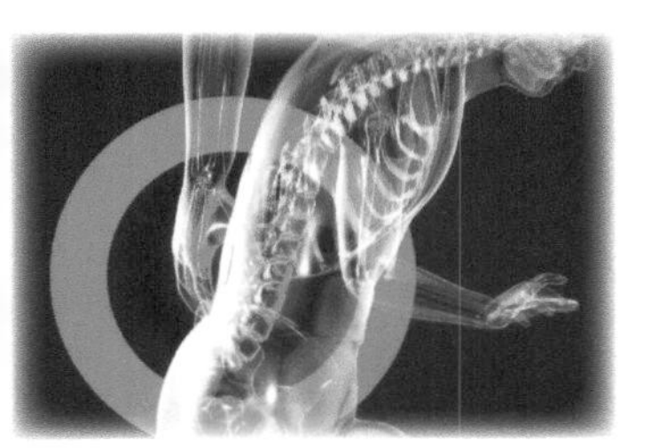

The spine should be treated as a whole unit. The treating healthcare provider must be cognizant of the fact that when one part of the spine becomes affected by a certain disease process and begins to generate pain, sooner or later, a "domino" effect will follow, affecting other articulating parts and complicating matters diagnostically and therapeutically. In essence, there is not one part of the spine that is totally spared following an injury or chronic mechanical stress. After all, the spine is a series of bones, one on top of the other, with overlapping neural innervations. It is not a solid biologic pillar, like long bones, such as the humerus and femur.

The diagnostic aspects of the majority of medical disorders are, for the most part, well-elucidated and established. Various therapeutic approaches to these disorders are fairly uniform, with very little variation in most clinics or hospital facilities. This is also true when it comes to conditions that require surgery, regardless of the location of the organ pathology. However, this is not the case in dealing with disorders of the mechanics of the spine, along with associated symptoms that are mediated by the various sensory innervations of the spine, including the nerve roots and fibrous structures that surround it.[60] Unlike soft tissue organs, the spine is a complex biological fibro-cartilaginous-bony structure that is well intricately engineered dating back to early embryological development. Perhaps this complexity, along with shouldering the full brunt of responsibility that it carries to support the entire body, are the reasons why the spine should be treated differently and cautiously. There is no single proven treatment that is superior or more effective than others for LBP; hence, the multiplicity of available treatment options.[75,76] It is literally the "backbone" of all daily living activities among humans, unlike coelenterates or members of the spineless lower phyla of the animal kingdom whose locomotion does not require the presence of a spine.

Since several structures in the spine can be affected or injured by alterations in its biomechanics at any one time following an injury or chronic poor posture, it is not surprising that treatment failure is more than likely to occur. The use of discography, facet block injection, and SPECT scans is helpful, but a positive result does not necessarily lead to definitive and effective therapy. False-positive results have been reported in facet joint injections and other diagnostic procedures.

The most conservative form of therapy consisting of rest, anti-inflammatory medications, and physical therapy (see commentaries on physical therapy in Chapter 7) is preferred by patients who have reservations about surgery.[Online9] Some prefer chiropractic therapy or osteopathic medicine. If spinal injections can localize the generator of pain, delivery of the medication to the source of pain can relieve the pain temporarily. Pharmacologic interventions[25] usually consist of nonsteroidal anti-inflammatory medications, most of which are available over the counter in all drugstores and are either taken orally or applied topically—acetaminophen, and nonbenzodiazepine muscle relaxants (carisoprodol, methocarbamol, tizanidine, and baclofen). Opioids, even short-term intake, can lead to dependence. Marijuana is increasingly used for the treatment of several neurological disorders characterized by pain and spasticity, such as multiple sclerosis and some spinal cord disorders. Several states in the U.S. have approved it for medicinal use. However, the chronic use of marijuana can induce aggressive and violent behavior and complicate matters medically and legally. Cannabidiol,[58] more commonly known as CBD oil, is available without prescription, but it is expensive. In two case reports, the use of levodopa was found to be beneficial for LBP associated with restless legs.[117]

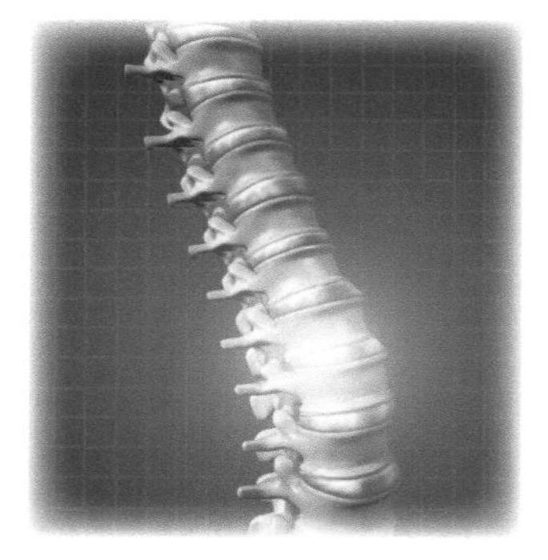

For radicular pain, epidural steroid injections may provide diagnostic (identification of pain generator) and therapeutic (immediate relief of pain) benefits. The injection can be repeated as needed, although the number of injections in a year has not been determined.[Online8] If a patient needs more than four in one year, surgery may have to be considered (a consensus statement by the North American Spine Society.[online 33,34]

Lumbar stenosis is a prevalent and frequent cause of low LBP and leg pain in older adults [57,77] The pain exacerbates when walking (neurogenic claudication). It can mimic leg pain related to arterial insufficiency (vascular claudication). A CAT scan is the preferred test procedure for diagnosis. As first-line therapy, it is treated with physical therapy, modification of physical activity, and judicious use of oral analgesics. Although epidural steroid injections can be beneficial in acute exacerbations, long-term benefits have not been established. Decompressive surgery has been recommended as a last-resort procedure, but with variable results. This variation is not unexpected because of the frequent concurrence of spondylolisthesis, facet joint inflammation, and multiple discopathies, which may require a different or more extensive surgical approach.

Not uncommonly, sacroiliac (SI) joint irritation can occur and can be overlooked during the course of treatment for LBP. The pain can mimic pain from primary spinal pathology, but local tenderness over the SI is diagnostic. Diagnostic and therapeutic injections of this joint can provide substantial pain relief. Injury and arthritis are frequent causes of SI irritation, and they can be irritated during or following pregnancy. The joint may become compromised when it compensates for chronic discopathies and facet joint inflammation. These concurrences attest to the complexity of the biomechanics of the spine, along with an almost unavoidable "domino" effect initiated by an injury to one particular joint or disk. Radiofrequency denervation has been used to treat SI joint and facet joint pain with variable results.[56]

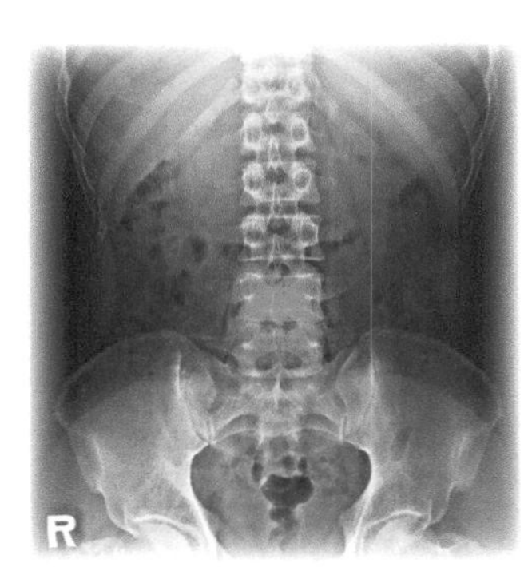

The zygapophyseal joints, more commonly known as facet joints, whose neural innervations have been well established, have been the focus of attention by pain interventionists. Irritation of the joints has been implicated in the majority of patients with LBP. Good knowledge of the innervations of the joints is crucial to successful injection therapy. These joints are innervated by the medial branch of the dorsal primary ramus, with each one receiving innervations from the medial branch at that level and the one above it. Despite well-established innervations, the therapeutic role of injection therapy remains controversial, leaving some investigators to question the condition as a distinct clinical entity. Treatment of facet joint syndrome includes intra-articular injections, medial branch blocks, and radiofrequency neurotomy.[95,112] Some have used intra-articular injections with autologous platelet-rich plasma with success and pain relief lasting for three months.[114]

For those with painful and spastic paraspinal muscles, Botox injection may provide significant relief. Botox is a neurotoxin produced by the bacterium Clostridium Botulinum. It acts presynaptically by blocking the action of the neurotransmitter acetylcholine on the skeletal muscles. It is used to treat spasticity from various neurological disorders, facial wrinkles, excessive sweating, overactive urinary bladder, neuralgias, and migraine. It is quite expensive, and some insurance companies do not cover this expense. The FDA has yet to approve of its use for LBP.

Complications from spinal injection treatments are the result of needle placement and the administration of the medication. Infection, hemorrhage, nerve trauma, air embolism, inadvertent intravascular or subdural injection of medication, urinary retention, radiation exposure, trauma to the disk, and allergic reactions have been reported.[44] With strict asepsis and antisepsis, along with accurate needle placement, these complications are preventable.

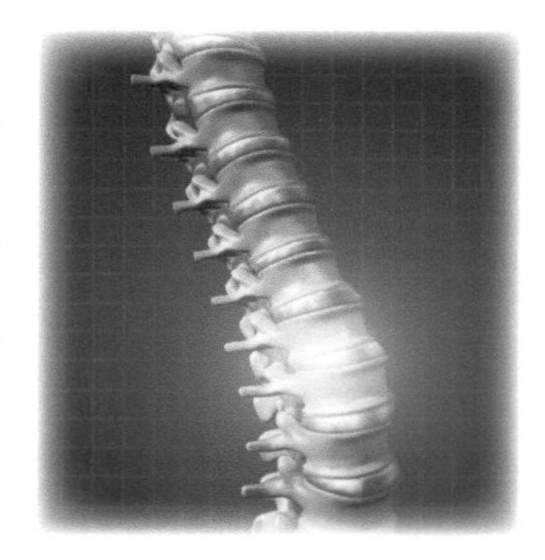

It is almost unavoidable to consider surgery for patients with unrelenting LBP who fail to obtain benefits from conservative treatment, including spinal adjustment and various spinal injections.[102] There are different types of low back surgery depending on the location of the target lesion that generates the pain. Surgery is either traditional (open approach) or minimally invasive—the former has a longer recovery time while the latter is less invasive and uses a tubular retractor to create a small tunnel that will lead to the surgical site. Recovery is for the latter. Traditional and minimally invasive spine surgeries include lumbar spine fusion, laminectomy or laminotomy, open diskectomy or microdiscectomy, foraminotomy, and artificial disk placement. There is no question that radicular deficits resolve dramatically following a diskectomy. However, subsequent studies have shown that many patients with lumbar disk herniation would improve without surgical intervention, hence the argument to institute conservative therapy first.

Depending on the nature of pathology in the spine—such as spinal deformities, spondylolisthesis, lumbar stenosis, instability due to severe arthritis, or after removal of an extruded disk—fusion using exogenous metal or bone (autograft or allograft) can be performed to stabilize the spine. Fusion was developed based on the principle that if pain occurs or aggravates in any position, it follows that stabilizing and immobilizing the spine by surgical interbody fusion will eliminate the pain. Fusion is accomplished using either an open technique or minimally invasive surgery, depending on the surgeon's experience. To access the spine, a posterior, anterior (abdominal), or lateral approach can be used, depending on the type and location of the fusion. Potential complications, as in any other surgery, include infection, poor wound healing, thrombosis, injury to blood vessels and nerves, and local pain from the source of the bone graft (usually the iliac crest of the pelvis). Patients should be aware that spine mobility will be greatly and permanently limited after fusion.

In recent years, the advent of laser therapy for lumbar disk disease has provided patients with minimally invasive surgical options that are helpful in reducing surgical risks and shortening hospital stays.49 If the source of pain can be pinpointed, laser disk decompression seems an attractive alternative to other forms of surgery. With the help of imaging technology, a small probe containing a laser is directed toward the affected disk. The energy generated by the laser removes the tissue impinging on the spinal nerve. Realistically, however, although it can relieve radicular pain, the relief of LBP may not necessarily follow.

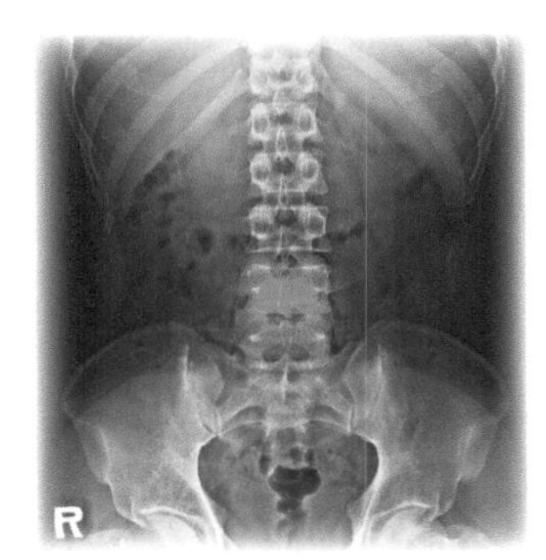

In the past, the use of chemonucleolysis with chymopapain offered hope to some patients and surgeons. Chymopapain is a nonspecific proteoglycanase enzyme derived from the papaya plant. When compared with the traditional approach, infection rates, hemorrhagic events, and neurologic deficits ere considerably lower with this procedure. Several years after it was introduced in the mid-sixties, the FDA approved the procedure. Its popularity, however, waned owing to reports of anaphylactic reactions, disk inflammation, subarachnoid hemorrhage, and various neurologic deficits, including myelitis. The procedure has no longer been in use since the 2000s. The discovery of other enzymes with less allergenic potential, like collagenase, may rejuvenate this procedure in the future.

In the real world of clinical practice, it is seldom that a physician encounters a simple or straightforward condition. This is the case when dealing with lumbar disk disease, especially after the age of twenty-five, when the disks begin to degenerate. The outer fibrous layer begins to weaken, slowly exposing the nucleus pulposus, making it likely to extrude following an injury. Between the ages of thirty-five and forty, LBP begins to occur. By the time the patient consults a healthcare provider following a back injury, a constellation of spinal abnormalities can be seen in radiographic studies. It then becomes quite challenging to determine the source of LBP. Spondylolisthesis, spondylolysis, facet joint inflammation, scoliosis, and various degrees of osteoporosis are, more often than not, seen concurrent with disk desiccation and/or herniation. Things become more problematic when the patient complains of various sensory or motor symptoms in the lower extremities and, in the worst situations, urinary bladder disturbances. When the latter symptoms are present, do they signify spinal root impingement, or are they referred from articulations in the spine or desiccated disk? Neurologically, the presence of typical dermatomal sensory deficits, focal motor weakness (foot drop, difficulty plantar flexing the foot or knee, and thigh instability), and changes in the reflexes are unequivocal signs of nerve root impairment. So, what is the next course of action.

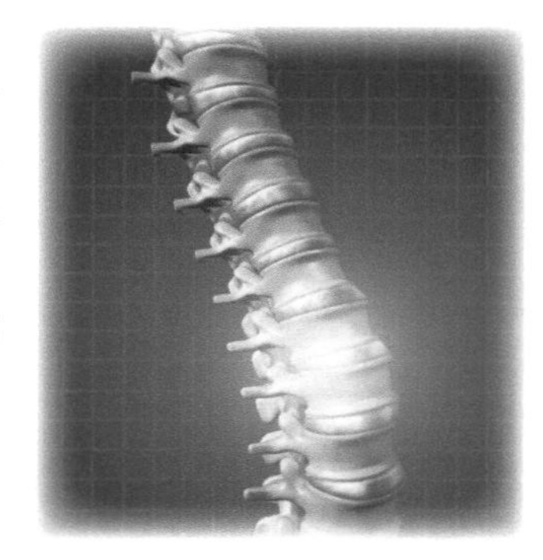

Most healthcare providers will proceed to rule out any systemic disorders that may be causally related to LBP. This is a prudent approach to patient management. When everything else is ruled out, the patient is either referred directly to a surgical specialist or for EMG and MRI (or CAT scan). A series of expensive diagnostic procedures then follow. If it is established that disk herniation is the main pathology, the following important questions must be answered: (1) What is the appropriate treatment for mild LBP with prominent signs of radiculopathy? (2) How about for a 50–50 pattern of LBP and radiculopathy? (3) How about for a severe LBP with questionable signs (or absence) of radiculopathy, clinically and/or electromyographically? If surgery is performed, the following hypothetical outcome can be expected, granting that all conservative measures are instituted. For question 1, the resolution of radicular symptoms, especially shooting pain, is immediate following a diskectomy. For question 2, radicular symptoms may improve after surgery, but LBP may persist. For question 3, LBP is likely to persist or worsen.

In the preceding discussion, it is evident that LBP and HD can be separate entities, but the two are likely to occur together following a spinal injury. For those with very disabling LBP with no neurologic or electromyographic abnormalities despite the presence of HD, it behooves the healthcare provider to look for other generator(s) of LBP. If no other causative generator of pain is identified, it can be argued that the SVN—those nerves that innervate the disks—are traumatized; hence, a possible justification to proceed to surgery while realizing that LBP may remain persistent owing to the unique overlapping and multisegmental distribution of the SVN (the Q2 and Q3 hypothetical outcomes outlined above).

Studies and anecdotal observations show that an untreated HD (even a large disk) may undergo spontaneous regression, and this has important therapeutic and prognostic implications.[14,27,43,59,72] This situation is relevant to the decision-making situation in patients with HD with LBP in the setting of the absence of neurologic deficits and EMG abnormalities. For most advocates—clinicians and surgeons—the treatment approach is conservative, even in the presence of radicular symptoms. However, it should be noted that early surgery may provide immediate relief from neurologic symptoms and, in some instances, relief from LBP.

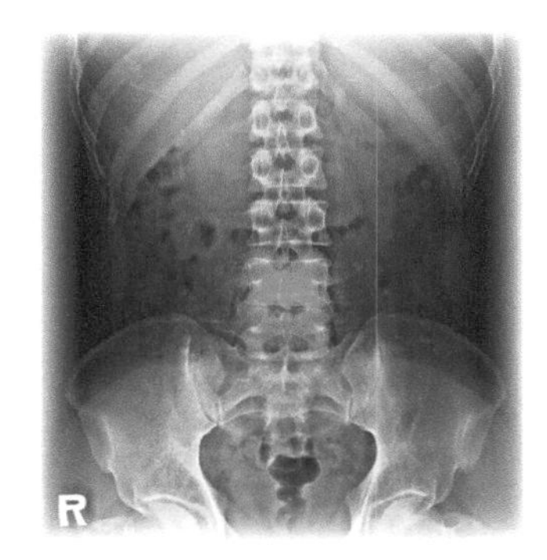

In recent years, lumbar disk replacement has been used in some medical centers to treat desiccated disks. An artificial disk usually consists of a combination of metal and plastic. The procedure is quite selective: it should be ascertained that the source of pain originates from one or two disks, there are no significant degenerative arthropathies, the patient must not be overweight, there is no spinal deformity, like scoliosis, and there is no previous surgery to the spine. Unfortunately, as in other surgeries, complications can occur, including infection around the disk, dislocation of the disk, and marked stiffness and rigidity of the spine. Technical and implant failure can lead to severe pain and loss of mobility.

As complications from low back surgery remain difficult to avoid, the quest for minimally invasive treatment of disk disease continues to evolve. Experimental studies using intradiscal injection of hyaluronan-methylcellulose hydrogels loaded with mesenchymal stromal cells into injury-induced intervertebral disk degeneration in Sprague-Dawley rats showed promising results. Injection of thermosensitive injectable glycol chitosan-based hydrogel into the porcine model induced effective filling of the degenerating disk. In one prospective human trial, injection of ethanol gel into the degenerating lumbar disk in sixty-seven patients who were followed for one year showed significant relief of both low back and radicular pain. With the patient sedated, injection of hydrogel is performed under fluoroscopic imaging.[16-18] Clinical trials are now underway in most major clinics in the world.[Online20,21]

In view of the inordinately high incidence of FLBSS, another minimally invasive technique to treat LBP from a degenerating disk involves stem cell implants.[82,Online27] The treatment process is still in its infantile stage, although advances and optimism have grown in the past ten years. The viability of the implanted cells (patient's own intervertebral disk, adipose tissues, or homologous cells) years after implantation remains an important issue. The technique of cell culture, delivery of the cells and instrumentation, proper patient selection and establishment of criteria, and precise localization of pain generator together with bureaucratic and health insurance issues constitute obstacles to its general acceptance in the treatment of discogenic LBP.

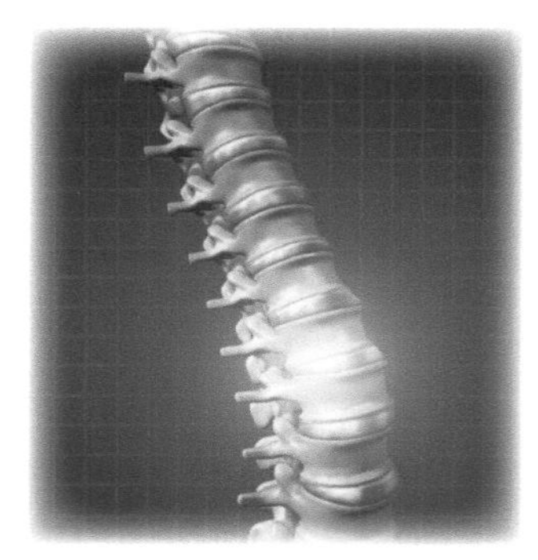

Foraminotomy is another surgical procedure that may be considered for spinal nerve impingement by a narrowed foramen, part of the spine where the spinal nerve exits.[1,34] The symptoms stemming from spinal root impingement in the foramen must be distinct, with clear clinical symptoms that correlate with the radiologic findings because foraminal stenosis can be asymptomatic. Moreover, it does not produce diffuse back pain, in contrast to discogenic pain. In this situation, conservative therapy is appropriate. Risks of foraminotomy include infection, injury to the nerve root, and recurrence of pain months or years after the procedure.

Surgery for non-disk-related LBP, as in facet syndrome, is an option if conservative measures (i.e., joint injection, nerve block and ablation, anti-inflammatory medications) prove ineffective.[95] The aim of surgery is to relieve pain, promote good mobility, and stabilize the spine.[30] Surgery is performed if a significant portion of the facet is fractured or displaced. In uncomplicated cases, a minimally invasive approach is the procedure of choice. Surgical fusion using bone grafts, rods, screws, and spacers stabilizes the spine. If there is a need to decompress the spine in facet disorders that lead to spondylolisthesis, a laminectomy may have to be performed to restore the space in the spinal column. The presence of bone spurs that may impinge on spinal nerves may require a facetectomy. Pathophysiologically speaking, it should be realized that regardless of the therapeutic modalities—conservative or surgical—the basic underlying arthropathic process will continue to persist even after surgery, and that all these treatments are merely designed to relieve the symptoms. They are not curative, and that is the reality that patients should know.

For some patients who, despite numerous interventional treatments, remain incapacitated by LBP, spinal cord stimulator implants may offer some partial pain relief. However, there are serious complications that patients must know. These include aggravation of the preexisting pain, paralysis, spinal fluid leak, spinal cord injury, bleeding, infection, pneumothorax and lung collapse, allergic reactions, and device displacement and failure.[Online10,11] Relief from transcutaneous nerve stimulation is minimal to moderate. Anecdotally, I have yet to see a patient who has benefited significantly from the implant.

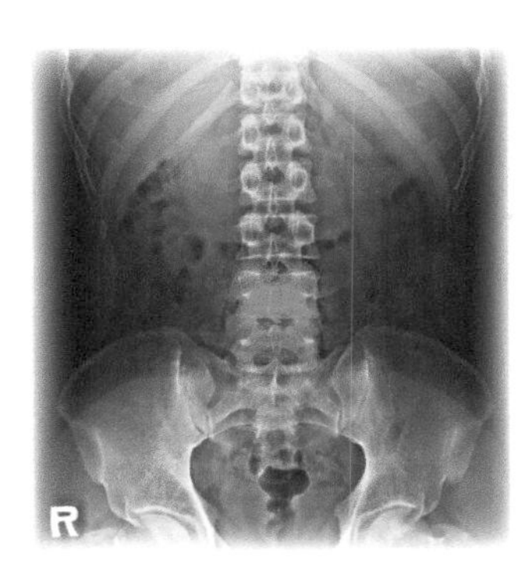

CHAPTER 7

Physical means to treat low back pain—Comments and opinions

Failure gave me strength.
Pain was my motivation.

—Michael Jordan, the greatest basketball player of all time.

Two barrels of tears will not heal a bruise.

—Chinese proverb

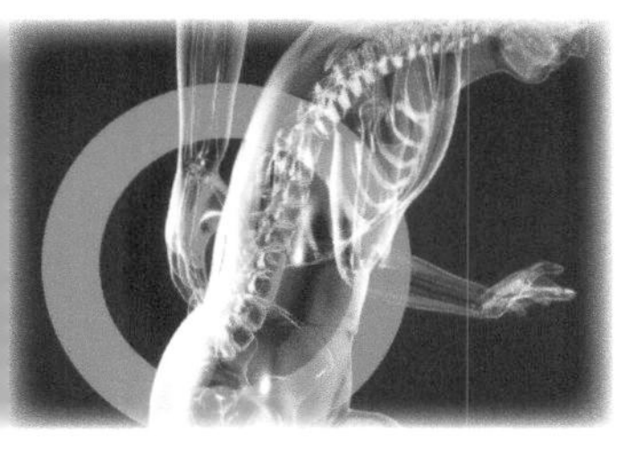

The treatment of LBP is quite challenging to all healthcare providers and is even more challenging when dealing with patients who fail to improve following surgery. No one therapy has proven to be superior to any other. The foregoing discussion about the complexity of the anatomy, physiology, and biochemistry of the spine provides some understanding of the mechanism of pain and its tendency to persist and perpetuate itself. The burden of supporting the entire body along with the complex anatomical structure of the vertebra that interplays with various chemical mediators of pain, the level of which increases following a certain injury, is quite phenomenal. In other organs, in general, when a pathology is identified, treatment is relatively straightforward, with few exceptions. This is not the case in the treatment of LBP or FLBSS. The inordinately high incidence of FLBSS and the failure of interventional therapy to offer significant and long-lasting relief from LBP brings to light the reality that the spine is truly special and unique. Hippocrates, a Greek scientist and father of Western medicine, remarked, "When in sickness, look to the spine first." When dealing with a patient with certain symptoms, such as pain, difficulty with locomotion, bladder disturbances, and impairment of sensory perception, it is indeed logical to look at the spine first, and then to other organs if the spine is found to be normal. However, it is clear that when a person complains of LBP, localization of pathology is straightforward, but applying appropriate therapy is another issue.

The surge of cytokines and various chemical mediators of pain following an injury to the lumbar spine can create a treatment dilemma when surgical intervention is considered to treat pain. Such biochemical phenomena can worsen theoretically during the course of surgical tissue manipulation. It is understandably justifiable to consider surgery when there are gross neurologic deficits or severe vertebral displacements and/or fractures, but if none of these exist, and if pain is the only prominent symptom in the setting of minimal laboratory abnormalities and an absence of neurological deficits, it is logical, based on our current knowledge of the spine, that the ideal treatment should be conservative. This is a situation in which the physical means of managing LBP is a safe and ideal approach. The ethical rule of modern medicine states, "First, do no harm."

Historically, the practice of using therapeutic movement therapy might have originated in China in 3000 BCE. Ancient physicians in Greece prescribed manual therapy and exercise to treat pain and certain diseases. Later, the Romans used movement exercises to rehabilitate injured soldiers of the Roman Empire. In ancient Japan and China, hydrotherapy was incorporated with physical exercise. The art of physical therapy in modern medicine took shape in Sweden in the eighteenth century, and it soon spread to most of northern Europe through the works of a group of British nurses. In the United States, women began administering massage and exercise therapy to soldiers of World War 1. In 1921, the American Women's Physical Therapeutic Association was founded by Mary McMillan and her fellow aides. This association is still operational.

Physical exercise for nonspecific LBP is recommended regularly by the Low Back Pain Guidelines. In addition, the use of other non-pharmacologic treatments, such as yoga, tai chi, massage, and spinal manipulation, are also recommended. For chronic LBP, physical therapy is the preferred first-line treatment of choice.[3,35,36,99,108]

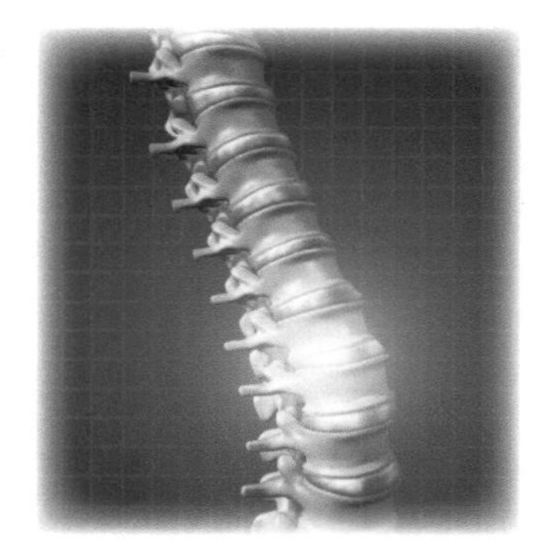

The management of acute LBP varies among physiatrists, osteopaths, general practitioners, and surgeons. Physiatrists tend to utilize physical therapy in acute cases of LBP. Rest and medications tend only to be associated with unfavorable outcomes, but incorporating some exercises may be beneficial. Given the variability in the treatment approach for acute LBP, it is always prudent, in the real world of clinical practice, to individualize therapy and not rely heavily on statistics. Moreover, no one particular physical exercise has proven to be superior to others.

Readers of this book who wish to know further details on how to perform back exercises are advised to read the references listed in the bibliography. In my experience, I find the application of physical treatments for patients with LBP favorable, but underutilized in some clinics. I should add that my experience with physical therapy as a patient with recurrent acute LBP is impressively favorable, with very little need for analgesics. LBP exercises recommended by the Mayo Clinic are quite useful.[Online22] They include flexibility exercises, stabilization exercises, and advanced stabilization exercises. The flexibility exercises include (1) single knee to chest, (2) lower trunk rotation stretch, (3) piriformis stretch, (4) double knees to chest, (5) hamstring stretch, (6) calf stretch, (7) hip flexor stretch, and (8) half kneel hip stretch. The stabilization exercises include (1) pelvic tilt, (2) pelvic tilt with legs, (3) pelvic tilt with arms, (4) pelvic tilt with bridging, (5) partial curl up, (6) standing pelvic tilt, (7) prone with leg raise, and (8) wall slides. The advanced stabilization exercises include (1) pelvic tilt with arms and legs, (2) pelvic tilt with straight leg raising, (3) bridging with straight leg raise, (4) all-fours with arms, (5) wall push-ups, (6) prone with arms/legs, (7) all-fours with arms/legs, and (8) half kneel to stand.

The role of standard chiropractic spinal adjustment in the treatment of LBP is well established. I refer select patients to chiropractors, particularly those without HDs, osteoporosis, or acute vertebral fractures. Patients with HDs, regardless of spine segment (cervical, thoracic, or lumbar), are referred to a physical therapist or physiatrist. The presence of two vertebral arteries inside the transverse processes of the cervical vertebra can be damaged by blunt trauma. Vertebral artery dissection leading to brainstem stroke are rare during spinal adjustment, but they can potentially occur. This complication is a catastrophic and life-threatening event. In the elderly, it is a bit risky to perform standard spinal adjustment, even in the absence of HD, because of the high incidence of degenerative osteoarthritis in the spine, which in itself can compromise the blood flow in the vertebral arteries. Rostrally, these arteries join to form the basilar artery, which supplies the brainstem and cerebellum, the posterior parts of the brain that regulate respiration, consciousness, sleep cycle, and coordination. Severe brainstem stroke resulting from vertebral artery injury is something to consider, especially in elderly individuals with preexisting atheromatous changes in the extracranial arteries (vertebrals and carotids).

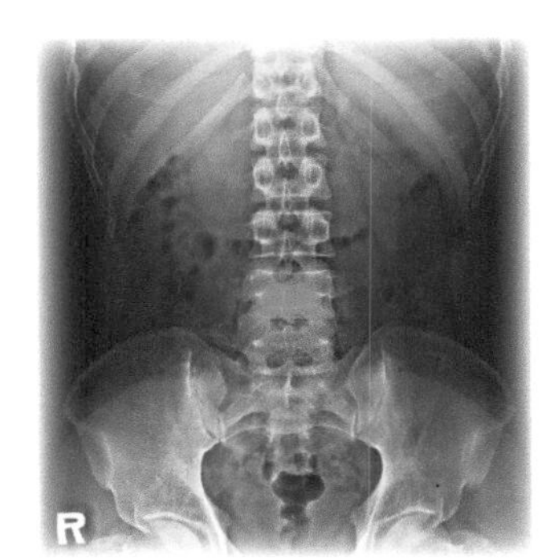

The presence of HD in the lumbar spine can be a risk factor for cauda equina syndrome, the occurrence of which can be facilitated by high-velocity spinal adjustment. This condition is due to compression of the lumbosacral nerve roots present at the end of the spinal cord. The nerve roots resemble the tail (cauda) of the horse (equine); hence, the term cauda equine syndrome. This condition is characterized by saddle anesthesia in the urogenital and anal areas and buttocks, urinary retention, sexual disturbances, and leg weakness. This is an urgent surgical condition. A case history is presented below.

A 60-year-old right-handed woman was referred for neurologic evaluation following a work-related injury. Shortly after the injury, she complained of severe LBP. The LBP extends vaguely to the thighs and legs. She was prescribed anti-inflammatory medication and referred by her primary care provider for physical therapy without significant improvement. Her medical history was essentially unremarkable. On neurological examination, I found her to have a significant degree of paraspinal muscle tenderness and spasm, along with limited anteroflexion of the lumbar spine. Furthermore, she had glove-stocking sensory deficits from the feet to the upper third of the legs. Her muscle stretch reflexes were hypoactive in the lower and upper extremities. Subsequent laboratory investigations revealed a protruded intervertebral disk at L4–5. The EMG showed no signs of active denervation, which correlated with normal strength. Interestingly, her nerve conduction examination demonstrated signs of sensory polyneuropathy (apparently asymptomatic at the time of the injury). Further inquiry revealed that there were two members in the family (her father and one son) with similar sensory symptoms and nerve conduction findings. Owing to her reluctance to undergo surgical evaluation, she elected to consult a chiropractor. Within a week, she presented to a local emergency room complaining of an inability to urinate and an inability to walk due to muscle weakness. She was later diagnosed with cauda equina syndrome secondary to a large lumbar herniated disc that subsequently required urgent surgery. She never recovered her baseline function and remained totally disabled, insofar as her original line of work was concerned. Her peripheral sensory neuropathy remained stable.

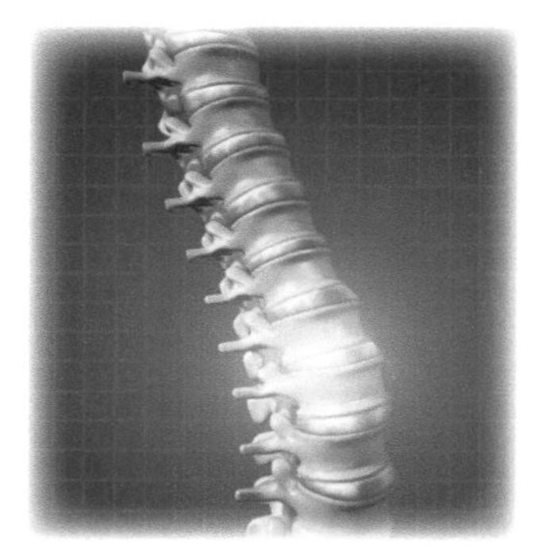

The causality between the worsening of her HD and spinal adjustment cannot be proven beyond a reasonable doubt or within a reasonable degree of medical certainty, but it cannot be totally ruled out.

CHAPTER 8

Biochemistry and immunochemistry of pain and the possibility that some cases of LBP may be a form of complex regional pain syndrome—Why do some patients continue to complain of pain even after successful surgery?

Pain of the little finger is felt by the whole body.

—Filipino proverb

Pain is inevitable; suffering is optional.

—Buddhist proverb

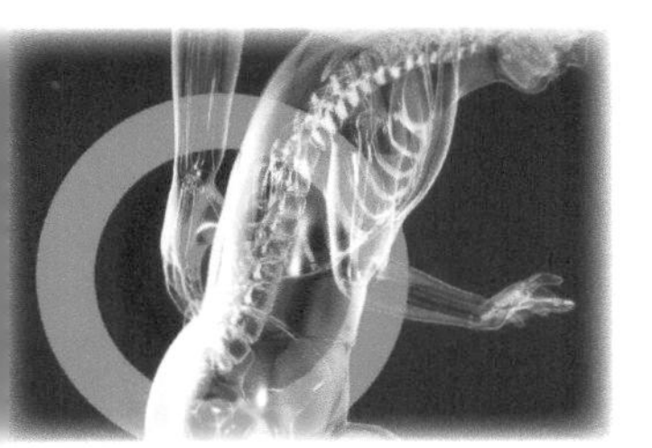

The search for effective treatment of persistent LBP, particularly the pain that persists despite the institution of various interventional and invasive surgeries, remains elusive. Given the complexity of the anatomical structure of the spine, together with several neurochemical mediators of pain that are released or activated following a certain injury or during an active phase of a degenerative process, it is not surprising to expect such distressing and unsettling situations for LBP sufferers. The medical, legal, and socioeconomic ramifications are obvious.

Persistent postoperative LBP, commonly known as "failed back surgery syndrome" is inordinately common and has been attributed to various preoperative and postoperative anatomical and mechanical factors in the spine. FLBSS may be associated with sensory symptoms in the lower extremities with or without EMG abnormalities. These sensory symptoms are frequently interpreted as radicular symptoms, which implies that the spinal nerve root is affected. It was brought up in one observational study that these sensory symptoms—those that are not associated with clear sensory loss, changes in the reflexes, and focal muscle weakness along with normal EMG—are actually pseudoradiculopathy. In addition, patients who complain of vasomotor symptoms in the lower extremities are also likely to suffer from persistent LBP, especially when the axial pain is quite severe and out of proportion to "radicular" symptoms. In this situation, if surgery is performed to include "decompression" of nerve root(s) in the absence of true radicular pathology, the outcome may not be favorable.

Numerous factors are implicated or associated with FLBSS; hence, the reasons why the term is ambiguous, imprecise, and misleading. There appears to be some unanimity in opinion among healthcare providers that a large number of patients with worker compensation claims evaluated for LBP or FLBSS are more likely to suffer from psychosocial issues (depression and anxiety) and persistent pain, or poorer outcomes after surgery. Although such an impression or perception may be valid, one cannot ignore the fact that people with workers' compensation claims have significant LBP. It can also be argued that depression and anxiety are merely secondary to LBP, frustration, and an inability to work. As alluded to in the foregoing discussion, there is a general consensus that surgery for LBP without signs of true radiculopathy has a higher rate of poor outcomes. Other factors include the presence of multilevel disk pathology, inflammation of facet joints, spondylolisthesis, spondylolysis, varying degree of spur formation, intra-operative and technical issues related to instrumentation, hematoma formation, infection, recurrent herniation, nerve injury, arachnoiditis, and epidural fibrosis.

Failure to recognize the presence of concurrent sensorimotor polyneuropathy can unfavorably affect the outcome of surgery. Polyneuropathy has a myriad etiology that generally includes familial inheritance, toxic-metabolic and systemic diseases, autoimmune disorders, vitamin deficiencies, and bacterial and viral infections. However, as much as 35% of those diagnosed with polyneuropathy have no identifiable etiology. A brief case history of a man with LBP and sensory-motor polyneuropathy is presented below.

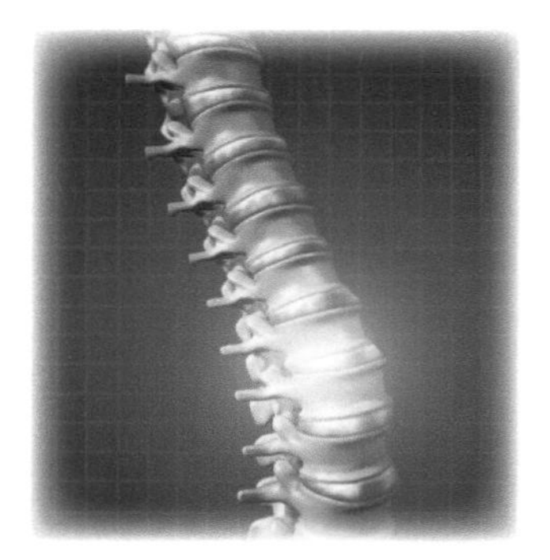

A 41-year-old man developed LBP following long-distance driving as a truck driver. The Workers' Compensation Board accepted his case as a work-related injury. The LBP was associated with bilateral foot drop and various sensory symptoms in the lower extremities, which he claimed he had never experienced before the injury. His medical history was otherwise unremarkable. Following a series of laboratory investigations, including a lumbar MRI, he was diagnosed with a moderate HD. He later underwent discectomy and laminectomy with autograft fusion at L4–5 without postoperative complications. He never improved, remained disabled, and continued to complain of LBP along with bilateral foot drop and paresthesias in the lower extremities. A subsequent nerve conduction examination revealed signs of mixed demyelinating and axonal polyneuropathy affecting the lower and upper extremities, along with signs of active denervation in the leg and foot muscles. In retrospect, this man's neurologic deficits were related to polyneuropathy and not to lumbar spine injury. This was a particular situation in which a neurologic examination elicited findings related to a separate issue and not to low back injury. A peripheral nerve conduction examination was clearly indicated owing to the presence of signs and symptoms of peripheral neuropathy. Otherwise, the procedure would have been noninformative or normal if those signs were absent.

To this day, it appears that the emphasis on the anatomical factors implicated in FLBSS remains the focus of attention of most surgeons. Therefore, the time has come to focus on the biochemistry and immunochemistry of LBP to provide alternative explanations for persistent post-operative LBP following uncomplicated and successful surgery, including FLBSS associated with various factors enumerated above.

Numerous studies have been conducted in recent years to determine the role of pro-inflammatory cytokines in acute and chronic persistent pain.[5,7,8,12,13,20,21,53,61,71,90,104,106,110,116,118] Cytokines are low molecular weight proteins secreted by cells of the immune system, and are produced during various inflammatory processes, including pain. They act as messengers between cells, and regulate the body's responses in both normal and pathologic states, such as infection, malignancy, and trauma. They include families of interferons, chemokines, tumor necrosis factors, interleukins and transforming growth factor, hematopoietins, and lymphokines. They are produced by various immune cells, such as B and T lymphocytes, macrophages, mast cells, endothelial cells, fibroblasts, and stromal cells. Recent studies have shown that patients with LBP have higher levels of proinflammatory cytokines compared with control subjects. This is unsurprising, since trauma can activate nociceptors, leading to the release of inflammation mediators, such as cytokines, bradykinin, and prostaglandins. Therefore, it is logically possible that additional trauma, including extensive tissue manipulation during surgery, may cause a surge in cytokines and lead to the perpetuation of pain. In such cases, would the use of monoclonal antibodies be effective in treating the pain of FLBSS? Therapeutic trials are currently underway.[92]

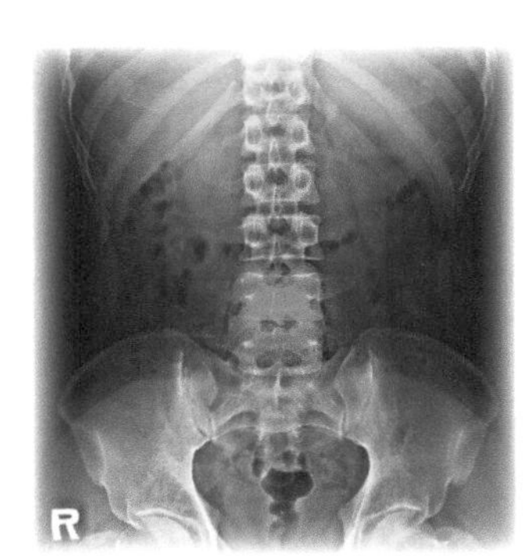

The unique anatomical system of the SVN innervations of the lumbar intervertebral disks may be relevant to PLBP. The multisegmental levels and overlap of disk innervations are responsible for the diffuse nature of discogenic pain. Therefore, localization of discogenic pain via discography may not necessarily lead to effective treatment. In fact, preexisting LBP may worsen during surgical tissue manipulation.

The intervertebral disk is poorly innervated and supplied only by nociceptive and postganglionic sympathetic nerve fibers. However, during degenerative processes, the disk becomes densely innervated and neovascularized and worsens preexisting LBP.

This pain is mediated by molecules of neurotrophins, which regulate the density and distribution of nerve fibers in peripheral tissues.[42,47] Neurotrophins are a family of proteins belonging to a class of growth factors that transmit signals to neural tissues to grow and differentiate, and they play a role in the inflammatory process and pain transmission. The pain can be worsened by concurrent facet joint inflammation, which can sensitize the local mechanoreceptors into becoming pain afferents, resulting in discogenic pain.

The possibility that some cases of PLBP may be a form of proximal complex regional pain syndrome (CRPS) is worthy of consideration and investigation.[65,68] This condition is a "self-perpetuating" chronic pain that usually affects the distal segments of the upper or lower extremities; it is characterized by allodynia (hypersensitive skin) and symptoms of sympathetic nerve dysfunction (cold or warm sensations), focal sweating, swelling, and discoloration and, in some instances, trophic changes affecting the integument and joints of the affected extremity. This possibility may not necessarily be far-fetched, considering that discogenic, and even facet joint pain, is mediated by both sympathetic and somatic nerve fibers. Some clinicians who take care of LBP sufferers are familiar with the presence of allodynia in the lower back, which may sometimes be construed as symptom augmentation or malingering. The elevated blood levels of inflammatory monocytes (CD14+ and CD16+) along with the shift toward a pro-inflammatory cytokine profile, despite the normal innate cytokine profile in CRPS, would suggest a potential role of the immune system in the pathogenesis of chronic pain, including LBP. For this matter, when the nucleus pulposus—an avascular and immune-privileged part of the disk—becomes extruded into the epidural space, a cascade of autoimmune reactions develops. These reactions involve activation of the macrophages and monocytes to initiate resorption of the HD. During the healing process, new vessel formation (neovascularization) occurs together with the spread of sensory nerve endings into the inner layers of the annulus. In a severely desiccated disk, the sensory nerve fibers can extend to the nucleus pulposus—the physiological and anatomical basis of discogenic pain.

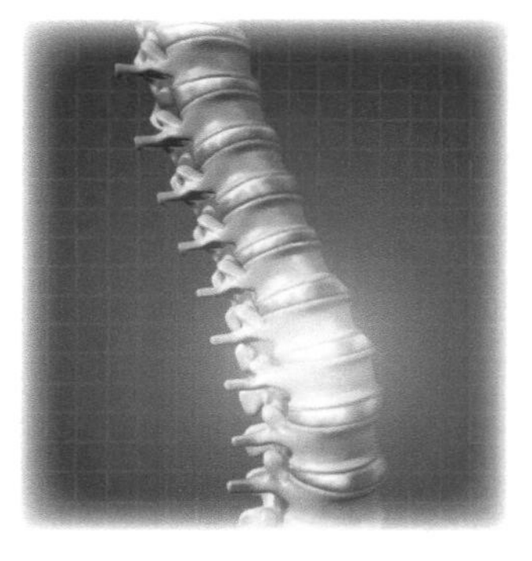

CHAPTER 9

Legal aspects and issue of disability

art of the problem with he word 'disabilities' is that t immediately suggests an nability to see or hear or walk r do other things that many f us take for granted. But vhat of people who can't feel?)r talk about their feelings?)r manage their feelings in onstructive ways? What of eople who aren't able to form lose and strong relationships? And people who cannot find ulfillment in their lives, or those vho have lost hope, who live in lisappointment and bitterness nd find in life no joy, no love? These, it seems to me, are the eal disabilities.

—Fred Rogers (1928–2003), The World According to Mister Rogers: Important Things to Remember.

The downside of my celebrity s that I cannot go anywhere n the world without being ecognized. It is not enough for ne to wear dark glasses and a wig. The wheelchair gives me away.

—Stephen Hawking (1942–2018), British theoretical physicist and cosmologist

When a person sustains a work-related injury to the lower back, the ensuing burdensome and usually protracted legal process can be a "backbreaking" experience, literally. Not only will that person suffer from the aggravation of and being subjected to—more often than not—chronic LBP and numerous diagnostic tests, but he or she will also have to deal with several members of the health care profession (i.e., a clinician, orthopedic surgeon or neurosurgeon, pain management specialist, physical therapist or physiatrist, psychologist, psychiatrist, and chiropractor), members of the legal profession (i.e., workers' compensation lawyer and lawyer representing the state insurance companies), an "independent" medical examiner, and members of the court system. The difficult task of presenting objective evidence to prove the validity of LBP stemming from a work-related accident can be arduous, frustrating, and emotionally distressing. There is a general perception among some doctors and laypersons that a patient injured at work is a malingerer seeking compensation, or someone who tries to augment or even fabricate the symptoms. Such a perception is the product of portrayal of some injured and disabled persons who were caught on TV surveillance cameras doing things that an ordinary disabled person is unable to do. Thus, bias against the injured becomes unavoidable. In my opinion, however, a great majority of them truly suffer from pain and must be given the proper attention they deserve.

It should be noted that there are other tissues that are not necessarily part of the spinal column that can be injured following a low back injury. Torn muscles, strained ligaments, and myofascial tissue disruption can cause long-lasting LBP. Some of these patients may not have demonstrable structural vertebral injuries or significant disk displacement, and yet the pain originating from those soft tissue injuries can be equally debilitating. Unfortunately, some patients with no demonstrable vertebral injuries or traumatic discopathies are often treated differently and unfairly. The trauma to these soft tissues may result in chronic pain and affect the amount of monetary compensation the injured deserve. Objective findings that correlate with the presence of soft tissue injuries can be demonstrated by infrared thermal imaging. They are seen as focal hot spots that are reproducible. Regardless, soft tissue injuries are frequently taken lightly by both sides of the legal panel—prosecution and defense—in contrast to spine injuries.

Most states require employers to provide employees with health insurance to cover the expenses for injuries sustained at work. They can get it either from state insurance funds or private insurers. The federal government has its own health insurance for its employees. The insurance company provides legal representation for the employer and provides protection for most lawsuits for on-the-job injuries or illnesses. After an injury, the worker is required to fill out questionnaires that include the date of injury, the name of the healthcare provider, lost wages and medical bills, and the name of the lawyer representing the injured. For healthcare providers, ordering a test procedure can be irritatingly inconvenient. Authorization from the state insurance carrier, especially for expensive tests such as MRI, CAT scan, SPECT, discography, myelography, and EMG, must be obtained before the injured person is evaluated. This may take several days or weeks. At times, the provider needs to discuss the necessity for certain test procedures with the so-called expert representative of the insurance carrier, who has not even seen or examined the injured employee. In the meantime, the injured individual continues to complain of pain and is forced to take potent narcotic analgesics or resort to taking herbal products and unproven treatments. When a test procedure like MRI is approved, there is usually a waiting period of days or weeks before it is performed. When the test report becomes available, the patient returns to the healthcare clinic to discuss the test results. When the results show equivocal or only mild findings, the patient will be informed that there is nothing serious and that he or she can go back to work. If the pain threshold of that injured individual happens to be low, and if there is a preexisting psychological issue, it may result in further aggravation of pain, which, in turn, may create doubt in the validity of the claim. Such a scenario will generate more arguments and legal maneuvering between the injured, together with his or her lawyer and the party representing the state insurance carrier. In search of more objective findings that will explain the pain and various symptoms associated with pain, members of the injured party may resort to ordering other diagnostic test procedures to support their claims.

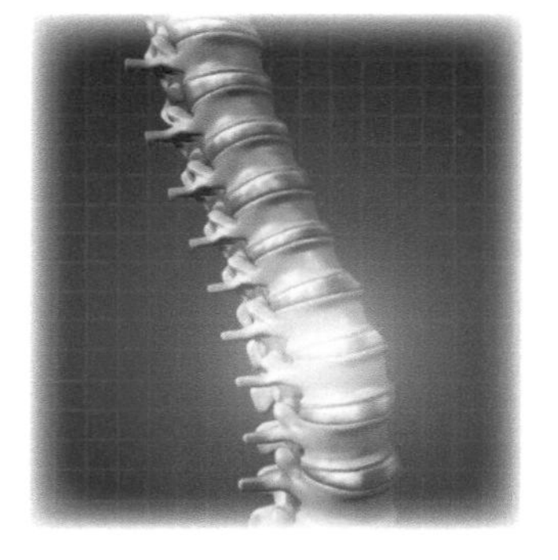

At some point during the process of evaluating and treating the injured, the claimant is frequently referred to an "independent" medical examiner, usually a physician, surgeon, or a chiropractor, who is typically hired by the insurance company. Most of the time, their opinions contradict or disagree with those of the treating healthcare provider. Many agree that they are not really independent. Their consultation fees may range from several hundred dollars to several thousand dollars for an average thirty-minute examination. Some of these examiners travel from one city to another (like a hired "gun") and write long reports (usually four to five pages long). The claimant may request that the examiner allow a relative or friend to witness the examination. Abnormal diagnostic test findings elicited by the treating physician are sometimes downplayed, and some may omit important findings that are favorable to the patient's claim. Such is the nature of the game played in workers' compensation cases. If necessary, the treating physician or surgeon will be deposed to present their opinions. The degree of disability of the injured and the permanency of the injury are presented. The judgment of the degree of disability can be controversial. Obviously, the more severe the disability, the higher the compensation award given on behalf of the injured, and the patient must be aware that every move or activity that he or she performs outside the house can be videotaped while the case is being controverted. This process of "spying" is routine and allowed by the court. The advice for patients is to act as naturally as possible or to do things commensurate with the level of disability or suffering—in other words, act properly. Otherwise, any physical activities disproportionate to the alleged level of disability can be used against the claimant.

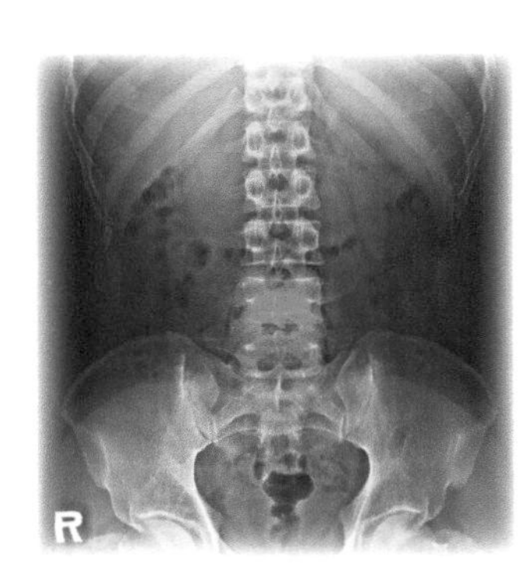

Some "diagnostic" clinics in some states solicit cases or offer services to injured workers and their legal representatives by performing tests that may validate the existence of injury-related symptoms. The most common symptoms in accident-related cases are pain, along with various symptoms such as tingling, numbness, and cold and warm sensations in the back and/or extremities. One particular test procedure is thermal imaging, also called thermology or thermography. For those who are unfamiliar with the technique of the science of thermology, it is often labeled as "voodoo medicine" by the uninformed. In reality, it is a sensitive, totally non-invasive, and painless test that measures the temperature and infrared heat emanating from the site of pain. It also provides objective documentation of cold temperatures in the limb affected by complex regional pain syndrome. In other words, it provides a "picture" of the manifestations of pain or sympathetic nerve activity. The temptation to use this test in all patients suffering from pain can lead to misuse and abuse of the procedure. One must realize that thermal imaging cannot quantitate pain, nor can it provide prognostication of a disease process. Moreover, it does not stand alone as a diagnostic test procedure. Few insurance companies cover the expense of this procedure, and because of the "bum rap" that it has received from many advocates of other test procedures, its popularity in the diagnosis of LBP has waned in recent years.

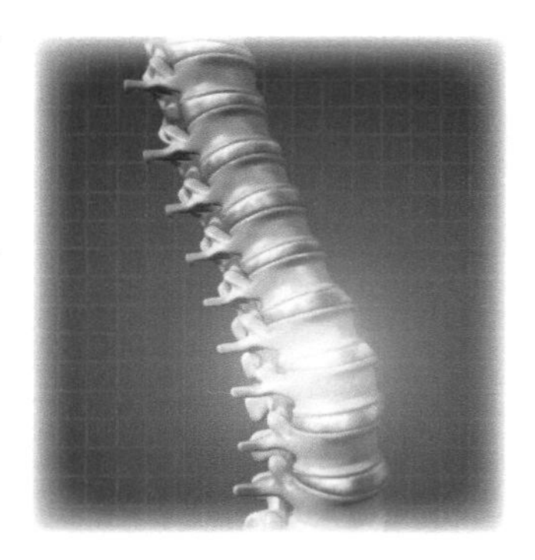

One disturbing aspect of some approved diagnostic test procedures is their ability to demonstrate certain "abnormal" findings that do not have clinical correlation at all. In essence, they are considered false-positive findings. The consequences are obvious. EMG, which is frequently performed in cases of LBP, can yield confusing results. Some electromyographers may report findings such as "polyphasic units" without other signs of active denervation and write a report to state that the findings are suggestive of some type of "radiculopathy." As stated previously, EMG can only assess the motor fiber components of the spinal nerve roots, and it cannot assess pain directly, particularly LBP, in the setting of a normal neurological examination. The various healthcare specialists who perform this procedure, each with varying degrees of neurological knowledge, make it difficult to obtain a uniform interpretation of the EMG results. This is a disconcerting aspect of EMG.

There is very little argument as to whether a certain test procedure that shows the presence of unequivocal pathology like HD has good clinical correlation, especially when associated with neurological deficits. However, in other instances, further test(s) may be necessary when LBP is out of proportion to HD with no associated neurological deficits. Healthcare providers with a good background in clinical neurology know full well that LBP and HD, even in the presence of radicular deficits, may not necessarily be mutually inclusive. For this matter, it behooves the treating physicians to consider looking for other cause(s) of LBP, such as facet joint inflammation or concurrent disk degeneration. In this situation, interventional therapy to treat the source of pain may have to be performed separately—or the source of pain and HD can be treated at the same time during surgery.

Most surgeons nowadays, unless there are severe neurologic deficits, as in cauda equina syndrome, would prefer conservative treatment, which is generally considered a prudent course of action. But how long the surgeon should wait before proceeding to surgery is an issue that needs to be addressed. If surgical intervention is performed early, will it prevent a "surge" of chemical pain mediators, or will it prevent neovascularization and activation of neurotrophins? If surgery is delayed, will it likely result in FLBSS for reasons stated in the foregoing discussion?

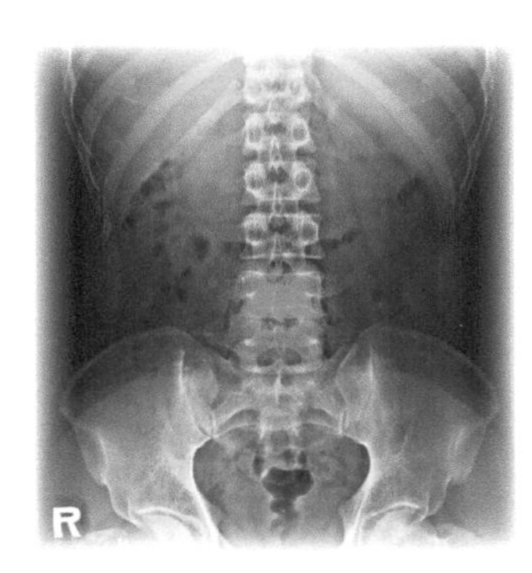

CHAPTER 10

What's on the horizon? Optimism and pessimism—The need to establish a "Dream Team"

When you have exhausted all possibilities, remember this: You haven't.

—Thomas Edison

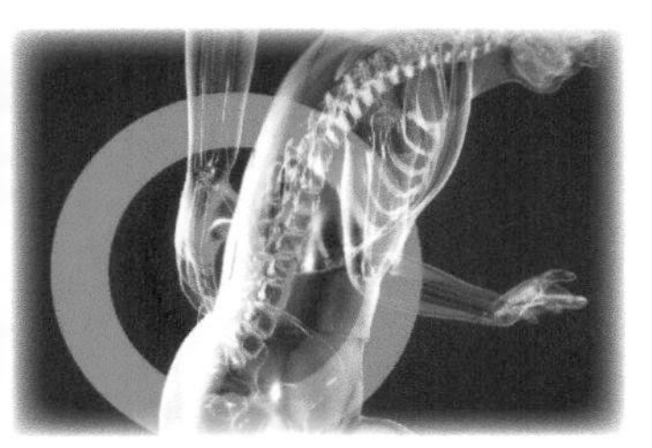

The formation of a team to formulate an ideal therapy for LBP sufferers can be logistically difficult, but not impossible. Ordinarily, when a patient is considered for surgery for LBP with or without radicular symptoms, the decision-making process is usually the surgeon's responsibility. The referring clinician, who receives a consultation note from a surgeon, is informed about the decision without any opposing or concordant views on the necessity for surgery from the referring clinician, physical therapist, or chiropractor. However, a decision-making process to determine the best option or course of action to take should ideally be made by a team, not by one person. Such an approach may have positive feedback from patients and relatives, regardless of the outcome of the surgical procedure. Given the controversies, a lack of uniformity in the diagnosis and treatment of LBP, and the high incidence of FLBSS, it is sensical that such a team effort approach be implemented. This is optimism.

Unfortunately, the tenacious adherence to certain treatment modalities by some healthcare providers, all armed with so-called scientific studies to support their practice guidelines, may provide obstacles to the formulation and application of certain diagnostic and/or therapeutic procedures. Some healthcare providers, particularly chiropractors, are traditionally opposed to surgery for LBP, with or without neurological symptoms. Some chiropractors, who have a background in the science of neurology, understand the indications for surgery in patients with neurologic deficits, particularly cauda equina syndrome or spinal cord compression. The lack of uniformity in the diagnostic and treatment approach to LBP, along with conflicts of interest and financial incentives on the part of practitioners, are, unfortunately, mightily difficult to overcome. This is pessimism.

The advent of multiple diagnostic procedures utilized in the evaluation of LBP along with multiple surgical techniques is a reflection of the complexity of the spine anatomy and physiology, and the ever-so-common FLBSS. The disinformation about the utility of certain test procedures contributes to the strain on healthcare costs, not to mention the tendency of some diagnosticians tout or overhype a test procedure. Thermal imaging, although effective in providing evidence for the existence of pain, does not play a crucial role in the overall management of LBP. EMG cannot assess pain directly, and it is uncomfortable and painful. An assessment of the F-wave and H-reflex is not cost effective and is useless in the setting of normal clinical examination. Realistically, what is the point of ordering the EMG procedure if there are no neurologic deficits. SEPs, unless there are signs of spinal cord compression and myelopathy, are useless in the evaluation of radiculopathies. A good clinical neurological examination can supersede these electrodiagnostic test procedures. However, not all LBP sufferers are seen by neurologists with expertise in the diagnosis of peripheral neurological disorders, such as those affecting the nerve roots, plexus, peripheral nerves, and skeletal muscles.

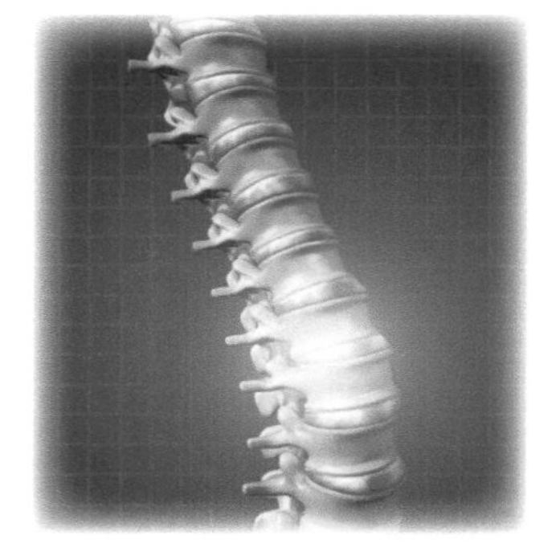

The discovery of pro-inflammatory cytokines, including a family of interferons, chemokines, tumor necrosis factor, interleukins, transforming growth factor, hematopoietins, and lymphokines—the systemic level of which increases in LBP—gave healthcare providers a deeper look at how pain is mediated and how it reaches the conscious level of awareness. The inflammation that results from extrusion of the disk and impingement of the nerve roots has been associated with the release of peptides such as substance P and bradykinin, calcitonin-gene related peptide, histamine, and phospholipase A, all of which have been implicated in the genesis of pain. Molecules of some members of neurotrophins belonging to a class nerve growth factor have been associated with an increase in fiber density in pain generated from disk degeneration. The identification of these chemical mediators of pain has paved the way to using monoclonal antibodies and nerve growth factor antagonists, a potentially novel pharmacologic treatment for LBP, or any other pain, for that matter. To overcome the shortcomings of conventional pharmacological agents, therapeutic trials are underway. The discovery of these pain mediators has led to the routine practice of administering calcitonin-gene-related monoclonal antibodies to migraine sufferers, either as a first-line treatment or for those who are unable to obtain relief from conventional therapy.

Tissue grafting, organ transplantation, and stem cell therapy are lumped together as forms of tissue engineering or regenerative medicine. In recent years, there has been growing interest in the use of stem cells for the treatment of LBP. Stem cells are also called undifferentiated master cells and can develop into several body organs. In contrast to monoclonal antibodies and anti-inflammatory drugs, which neutralize the effect of the chemical pain mediators that are released during inflammatory processes from disk disease and various joint inflammations, stem cell therapy offers definitive treatment. It has the potential to repair and restore the anatomy of a tissue or organ that has undergone years of degeneration, either through the aging process or repetitive physical stress exerted on the lumbar disks. Sources of stem cells are obtained from the embryonic inner cell mass of the blastocyst, placenta, umbilical cord, hematopoietic cells, bone marrow, and adipose-derived mesenchymal cells. In addition, stem cell therapy has shown promising results in the treatment of peripheral neuropathy, osteoarthritis, and various neuralgias. Because of the potential for the abuse and misuse of stem cell therapy, the FDA and Institutional Review Boards have been on top of these issues through strict regulations and oversights. Religious issues also have to be taken into consideration.

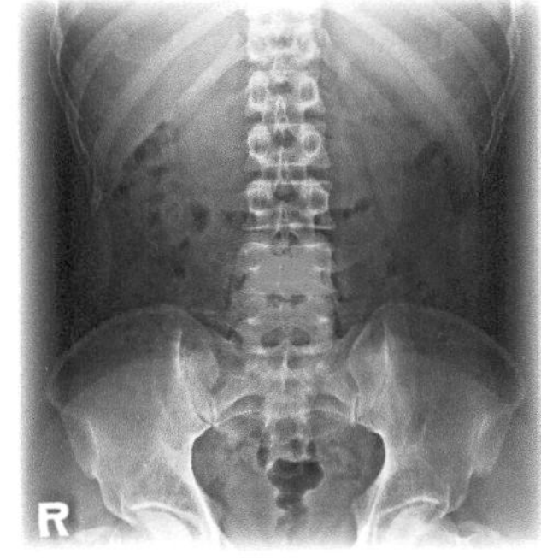

Pharmacology and nanotechnology have begun to intersect in the treatment of pain in recent years. Conventionally, when drugs are delivered to the site of the pain generator, side effects and adverse reactions are frequent, resulting from the effects of the drugs on other organs and tissues. The use of nanoparticles to deliver drug molecules specifically to the source of pain is an innovative way to circumvent these adverse reactions. As in other experimental treatment modalities, obstacles need to be overcome. These include determining the long-term effects of the nanoparticles and the expense of the treatment, together with proper patient selection and the establishment of criteria and contraindications. Although research on this subject is still in its infantile stage, the potential for clinical application of nanotechnology in pain management has arrived. Online31-32

CHAPTER 11

Recapitulation and thoughtful advice

Truth is the offspring of silence and meditation. I keep the subject constantly before me and wait till the first dawnings open slowly, by little and little, into a full clear light.

—Sir Isaac Newton (1642–1727), English mathematician, physicist, and astronomer

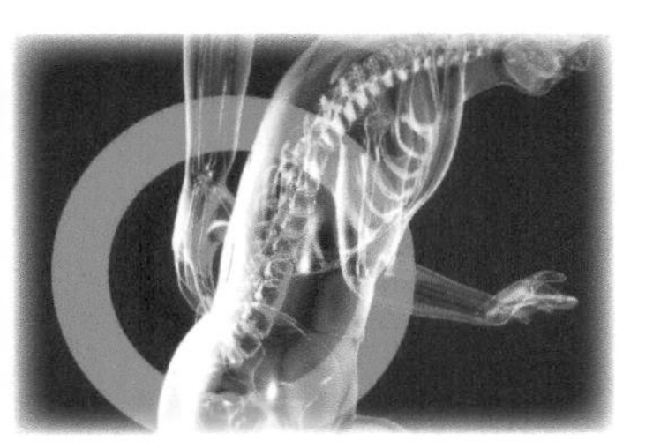

Regardless of what side of the fence you are sitting on—evolution or intelligent intervention—biped animals belonging to the phylum Chordata will always put strain on their vertebrae throughout their lifetime. The column of bones, stacked one on top of each other and protected by a cushion made of collagenous protein and water between each complex bony structure, is richly supplied by numerous blood vessels and pain-sensitive nerves (except nucleus pulposus), all designed to provide nutrition and to serve as sensors to detect any anatomical displacement of all articulating parts.

The nerve fibers that carry the pain sensation in the spine have an overlapping distribution that extends above and below each vertebra. This anatomical arrangement makes localization of the source of pain difficult. If a certain part of the spine is "ascertained" to be the source of pain, pain relief using invasive interventional procedures does not necessarily follow. A similar outcome can be expected from surgical intervention.

Radicular symptoms due to HD (shooting pain extending to the leg and foot, sensory loss and focal, muscle weakness like foot drop) and LBP are two separate clinical entities. They may occur together following back injuries. Surgical removal of the disk may not necessarily relieve LBP.

Several diagnostic test procedures were discussed in the previous chapters. In summary, MRI or CAT scans combined with good clinical neurological examinations are most useful. For nonradicular LBP, SPECT scans and discograms are useful, but these procedures should be used judiciously, especially as discograms may accelerate disk degeneration.

The presence of "root impingement" demonstrated on CAT scans or MRI should not be taken at face value without neurological deficits. Such findings should not be considered indications for surgery. I recall one classmate, a retired physiatrist in Bay State, who herself had LBP. She disseminated information to her fellow alumni that she had L5 root impingement, as demonstrated by the MRI. However, despite her specialty, it was unclear whether the radiologic findings had unequivocal neurological correlations or sensory and motor deficits (true radiculopathy). It appeared that she was relying heavily on the MRI findings for the cause of her LBP, not realizing that true radiculopathy and LBP are separate pathophysiologic entities. Fortunately, she avoided surgery owing to her age and concurrent cerebrovascular disorder. One other classmate, a successful practicing internist and president of the Mount Rushmore State Medical Association, who presented one day with LBP with radiological evidence of foraminal L4 root impingement but without signs of true radiculopathy, avoided surgery by utilizing extensive physical therapy and exercises, together with an intake of anti-inflammatory medications. Years later, he remained relatively asymptomatic and continued to enjoy his golf swings.

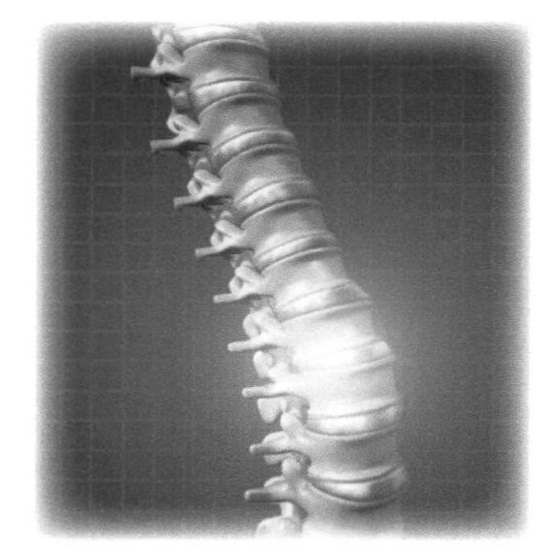

A CAT scan combined with a myelogram is useful in the evaluation of arachnoid disease, displaced nerve roots, metastatic cancer, lumbar stenosis, arthritis, and calcification of the posterior longitudinal ligaments.[100,113] It has been used infrequently in recent years due to the advent of MRI. A very bothersome complication is spinal fluid leak owing to a lumbar puncture, which can cause postural headaches, not to mention the great amount of radiation needed to do the procedure. Patients should be wary of serious complications from the use of contrast materials when undergoing CAT scans or MRI.

It is well accepted that EMG can localize the nerve root affected, but more often not, when neurologic deficits are already evident, clinical diagnosis will suffice with good clinical examination. Therefore, EMG is either optional or not indicated. Moreover, EMG can only assess the motor fiber components of the spinal nerves. It cannot assess pain directly, and it is a painful test procedure. It can be disconcerting to perform the procedure to someone already in pain. Likewise, SEPs cannot assess pain directly. They can only assess the large fibers—nerve fibers that do not carry pain impulses.

Thermal imaging is a useful and sensitive test for assessing the local vasomotor reactions associated with pain. It is totally painless, but it cannot quantify the severity of pain. Unfortunately, health insurance companies do not cover the expense. Bureaucratic issues prevent this procedure from being accepted as a valid diagnostic test procedure in the diagnosis of various pain syndromes.

All interventional treatments (spinal injections, Botox injections, various nerve blocks, and nerve ablations) are forms of symptomatic therapy. They do not cure the underlying disease. Injectable hydrogels are promising, but they are still another form of symptomatic therapy. Long-term efficacy remains to be seen. Intracept therapy that uses radiofrequency ablation of the basivertebral nerves (branches of the SVN that supply the vertebral end plates and disks) is quite promising[28-30] and is approved by the FDA.

LBP sufferers without HD, neurologic deficits, vertebral fractures, or significant osteoporosis are better off having spinal adjustments. Those with HD with neurologic deficits who wish to avoid surgery should undergo physical therapy.

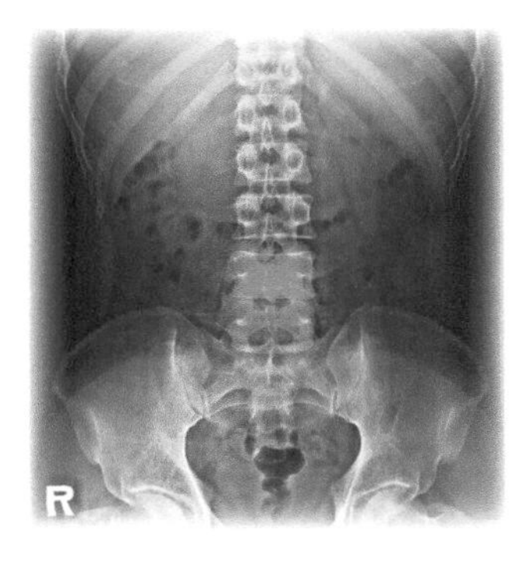

Patients diagnosed with FM and also suffering from LBP should seek the opinions of a neurologist to look for the possibility of SFN, a condition with several etiologies. Those with systemic symptoms, body malaise, loss of weight, and a history of alcohol abuse, drug addiction, and smoking should see an internist first.

In recent years, surgeries have been close to perfect and quite safe. Techniques are superb. Surgeons are very good at what they do. Realistically, all back surgeries are meant to stabilize the spine and relieve pain. Leg pain due to irritation of the nerve root(s) can be relieved by surgery quite significantly and dramatically, but it will not necessarily relieve LBP because neural innervations of the spine are separate and frequently overlap. Surgeries do not cure the underlying disease, but they can offer effective short-term, in some cases long-term, temporizing measures to improve the quality of life of LBP sufferers. Degenerative processes in the spine and disks, together with age-related bone loss, however, will continue and slowly progress after surgery. This is the reality.

Laser disk surgery and/or microdiscectomy are relatively less invasive and, in the hands of an experienced surgeon, can precisely remove the disk impinging on the spinal nerve. However, the presence of diffuse LBP that is associated with various and vague sensory symptoms, including cold and/or warm sensations in the lower extremities, may influence the outcome of surgery unfavorably. These symptoms are mediated by the sympathetic nerves, and can theoretically evolve and manifest as complex regional pain syndrome.[68]

It is well known that spinal fusion will diminish spine mobility. An artificial disk implant is an alternative to spinal fusion, but spine surgeons do not have clear guidelines regarding the timing of the implant. Clear indications have yet to be established. The complexity of the nerve supply of the lumbar spine has to be taken into serious consideration (note: always ask for a second or third opinion if surgery is being considered).

Stem cell implants or regenerative medicine are promising. It is now being used to treat various types of pain in joints. However, it is still considered experimental, so health insurance companies do not cover the expense. One of my patients with severe pain due to a degenerating lumbar disk who received stem cell therapy improved slowly but dramatically within a few months. The out-of-pocket expense was $5,000!

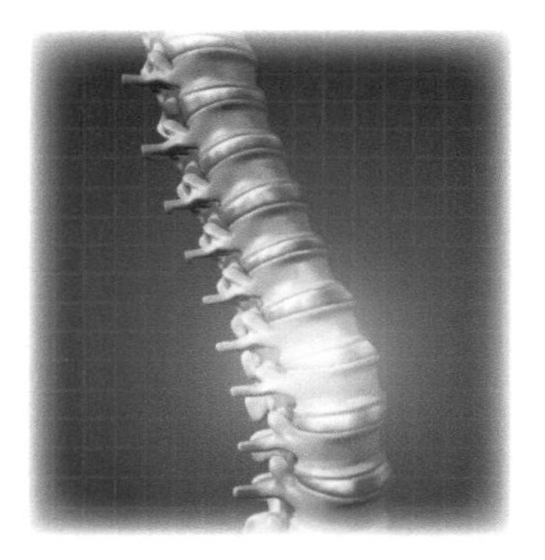

This is my personal opinion and recommendation. I think the decision to perform surgery (major or minimally invasive) for LBP sufferers should be a team effort—a cooperative and collaborative integration of various specialties. It makes sense to develop a "dream team" composed of a surgeon, neurologist, radiologist, pain management specialist, nurse and paramedical personnel, internist (with osteopathic expertise), physiatrist and physical therapist, psychologist, and even chiropractor to actively participate in the decision-making process. It may seem logistically difficult to organize such a team, but for the sake of openness, transparency, and sound medical practice, such an approach can be rewarding. It can yield favorable feedback from patients and relatives, regardless of the outcome of the surgery. This is optimism.

Finally, let me say that unless the exact pathogenesis of degenerative disk disease and various degenerative changes in the spinal articulations evolving and progressing in concert with the surge of various neurochemical mediators of pain become known and firmly established, all treatments for LBP, with or without true radiculopathy, will remain symptomatic forms of treatment. They are not curative but cure may soon light up the horizon as scientific advances are made.

BIBLIOGRAPHY

JOURNAL ARTICLES

1. Ahn Y, Oh HK, Kim H, et al. Percutaneous endoscopic lumbar foraminotomy: an advanced surgical technique and clinical outcomes. *Neurosurgery*. 2014;75"124-144.

2.Baber Z, Erdek MA. Failed back surgery: current perspective. *J Pain Res*. 2016;9:979-987.

3. Bahns C, Happe L, Thiel C, et al. Physical therapy for patients with low back pain in Germany: a survey of current practice. *BMC Musculoskelet Disord*. 2021;22:563. doi:1186/s12891-021-04422-2

4. Bartleson JD, Maus TP. Diagnostic and therapeutic spinal interventions: Discography. Neurol Clin Pract. 2014;4:353-357.

5. Benarroch EE. Dorsal horn circuitry: complexity and implications for mechanisms of neuropathic pain. *Neurology*. 2016;86:10160-1069.

6. Bordoni B, Marelli F. Failed back surgery syndrome: review and new hypothesis. *J Pain Res*. 2016:17-22.

7. Borish LC, Steinke JW. Cytokines and chemokines. *J Allergy Clin Immunol*. 2003;111(2 Suppl):S460-475.

8. Brenn D, Richter F, Schaible HG. Sensitization of unmyelinated sensory fibers of the joint nerve to mechanical stimuli by interleukin-6 in the rat: an inflammatory mechanism of joint pain. *Arthritis Rheum*. 2007;56:351-359.

9. Braun J, Baraliakos X, Kiltz U. Secukinumab (AIN457) in the treatment of ankylosing spondylitis. *Expert Opin Biol Ther*. 2016;16:711-722.

10. Brisson BA. Intervertebral disc disease in dogs. *Vet Clin North Am Small Pract*. 2010;40:829-858.

11. Carragee EJ, Don AS, Hurwitz EL, et al. Does discography cause accelerated progression of degeneration changes in the lumbar disc? A ten-year matched cohort study. *Spine*. 2009;34:2338-2345.

12. Cavanaugh JM, Ozaktay AC, Yamashita T, et al. Mechanisms of low back pain: a neurophysiologic and neuroanatomic study. *Clin Ortho Relat Res*. 1997;335:166-180.

13. Chiarotto A, Koes BW. Nonspecific low back pain. *N Engl J Med*. 2002;386:1732-1740.

14. Chiu CC, Chuang TY, Chang KH, et al. The probability of spontaneous regression of lumbar herniated disc: a systematic review. *Clin Rehabil*. 2015;2:184-195.

15. Chou R, Baisden J, Carragee EJ, et al. Surgery for low back pain: a review of the evidence for an American Pain Society Clinical Practice Guideline. *Spine*. 2009;34:1094-1099. doi:10.1097/BRS.ob13e318a105fc

16. Choi UY, Joshi HP, Payne S, et al. An injectable hyaluronan-methylcellulose (HAMC) hydrogel combined with Wharton's jelly-derived mesenchymal stromal cells (WJ-MSCs) promotes degenerative disc repair. *Int J Mol Sci*. 2020;21(19):7391. doi:10.3390/ijms21197391

17. Latka K, Kozlowska K, Waligora M, et al. Efficacy of discogel in treatment of degenerative disc disease: a prospective 1-year observation of 67 patients. *Brain Sc.* 2021;11(11)1434. doi.10.3390/brainsc11111434

18. Li Z, Shim H, Cho MO, et al. Thermo-sensitive injectable glycol chitosan-based hydrogel for treatment of degenerative dis disease. *Carbohydr Polym.* 2018;184:342-353. doi:10.1016/j.carbpol.2018.01.006

19. Christellis N, Simpson B, Russo M, et al. Persistent spinal pain syndrome: a proposal for failed back surgery syndrome. *Pain Med.* 2021;4:807-818.

20. Cuellar JM, Golish SR, Reuter MW, et al. Cytokine evaluation in individuals with low back pain using discographic lavage. *Spine J* 2010;3:21-218.

21. Cunha C, Silva AJ, Pereira P, et al. The inflammatory response in the regression of lumbar disc herniation. *Arthritis Research & Therapy.* 2018;20:251. doi:1186/s13075-018-1743-4

22. Daly C, Ghosh, Jenkin G, et al. A review of the animal models of intervertebral disc degeneration: pathophysiology, regeneration, and translation to the clinic. *Biomed Res Int.* 2016:5952165. doi:10.1155/20/2016/5952165

23. Daniell JR, Osti OL. Failed back surgery syndrome: a review article. *Asian Spine J.* 2018;2:371-379.

24. Delito A, George SZ, Van Dillen L, et al. Low back pain. *J Orthop Sports Phys Ther.* 2012;42:A1-57.

25. Deyo RA. Drug therapy for back pain: which drugs help which patients? *Spine.* 1996;21:2840-2850

26. De Maeseneer M, Lenchik L, Everaert H, et al. Evaluation of lower back pain with bone scintigraphy and SPECT. *Radiographics.* 1999;19:901-912.

27. Deyo RA, Mirza SK. Herniated lumbar intervertebral disk. *N Engl J Med.* 2016;374:1763-1772.

28. Diamandopoulos AA, Goudas CP. Human and ape: the legend, the history and the DNA. *Hippokratia.* 2007;11:92-94.

29. Dolan AL, Ryan PJ, Arden NK, et al. The value of SPECT scans in identifying back pain likely to benefit from facet joint injection. *Br L Rheumatol.* 1996;12:1269-1273.

30. Dreyfuss PH, Dreyer SJ, Herring SA. Lumbar zygapophysial (facet) joint injections. *Spine.* 1995;20:2040-2047.

31. Dudli S, Liebenberg E, Magnitsky S, et al. Modic type 1 change is an autoimmune response that requires a proinflammatory milieu provided by the "Modic disc." *Spine J.* 2018;18:831-844. doi: 10.10.1016/J spine.2017.12.004

32. Edgar MA. The nerve supply of the lumbar intervertebral disc. *J Bone Joint Surg* (Br). 2007;89-B:1135-1139.

33. Ellenberger C. MR imaging of the low back syndrome. *Neurology.* 1994;44:594-600.

34. Evins A, Banu MA, Njoku I, et al. Endoscopic lumbar foraminotomy. *J Clin Neurosci.* 2015;22:730-734.

35. Fritz JM, Cleland JA, Speckman M, et al. Physical therapy for acute low back pain: associations with sybsequent healthcare costs. *Spine.* 2008;33:1800-1805.

36. Groenendijk JJ, Swinkels ICS, de Bakker D, et al. Physical therapy management of low back pain has changed. *Health Policy.* 2007;80:492-499.

37. Hallast P, Jobling MA. The Y chromosome of the great apes. *Hum Genet.* 2017;136:511-528. doi:10.1007/s00439-017-1769-8

38. Fan Y, Newman T, Linardopoulou E, et al. Gene content and function of the ancestral chromosome fusion site in human chromosomes 2q13 – 2q14.1 and paralogous regions. *Genome Res.* 2002;11:1663-1672. doi:1101/gr.338402

39. Freemont AJ. The cellular pathobiology of the degenerate intervertebral disc and discogenic back pain. *Rheumatology.* 2009;48:5-19.

40. Fritsch EW, Heisel J, Rupp S. The failed back surgery syndrome: reasons, intraoperative findings, and long-term results: a report of 182 operative treatments. *Spine.* 1996;21:626-633.

41. Gagnet P, Kern K, Andrews K, et al. Spondylolysis and spondylolisthesis: a review of the literature. *J Ortho.* 2018;15:404-407. doi:10.1016/j.jor.2018.03.008

42. Garcia-Cosamalon J, Del Valle ME, Calavia MG, et al. Intervertebral disc, sensory nerves and neurotrophins: who is who in discogenic pain. *Journal of Anatomy.* 2017;217:1-15.

43. Gao S, Geng X, Fang Q. Spontaneous disappearance of large lumbar disc herniation. *JAMA Neurology.* 2018;75:123-124.

44. Goodman BS, Posecion LW, Mallempati S, et al. Complications and pitfalls of lumbar interlaminar and transforamial epidural injections. *Curr Rev Musculoskelet Med.* 2008;3-4:212-222. doi:10.1007/s12178-008-9035-2

45. Gore M, Sadosky A, Stacey BR, et al. The burden of chronic low back pain: clinical comorbidities, treatment patterns, and health care costs in usual care settings. *Spine.* 2012;37:e668-677.

46. Groen GJ, Baljet B, Drukker J. Nerves and nerve plexuses of the human vertebral column. *Am J Anat.* 1990;188:282-296.

47. Gruber HE, Hoelscher GL, Ingram JA, et al. Genome-wide analysis of pain-, nerve- and neurotrophin - related gene expression in the degenerating human annulus. *Molecular Pain.* 2012;8:63.

48. Hegmann KT, Travis R, Belcourt RM, et al. Diagnostic tests for low back disorders. *J Occup Environ Med.* 2019;61:e155-e168.

49. Hosseini B, Allameh F. Laser therapy in lumbar disc surgery – a narrative. *J Lasers Med Sci.* 2020;11:390-394.

50. Hoy D, March L, Brooks P, et al. The global burden of low back pain: estimates from the Global Burden of Disease 2010 study. *Ann Rheum Dis.* 2013;73:968-974.

51. Hughes JF, Skaletsky H, Pyntikova T, et al. Chimpanzee and human Y chromosomes are remarkably divergent in structure and gene content. *Nature.* 2010;463:536-539.

52. Inoue N, Espinoza Orias AA, Segami K. Biomechanics of the lumbar facet joint. *Spine Surg Relat Res.* 2019;4:1-7. doi:10.22603/ssrr.2019-1117

53. Jacobsen HE, Khan AN, Levine ME, et al. Severity of intervertebral disc herniation regulates cytokine and chemokine levels in patients with chronic radicular back pain. *Osteoarthritis Cartilage.* 2020;28(10):1341-1350. doi:10,1016/j.joca.2020.06.009

54. Jiang H, Moreau M, Raso VJ, et al. A comparison of spinal ligaments – differences between bipeds and quadrupeds. *J Anat.* 1995;187(Pt 1):85-91.

55. Jensen MC, Brant-Zawadzki MN, Obuchowski N, et al. Magnetic resonance imaging of the lumbar spine in people without back pain. *N Engl J Med.* 1994;331:69-73.

56. Juch JNS, Maas ET, Ostelo RWJG, et al. Effect of radiofrequency denervation on pain intensity among patients with chronic low back pain: the Mint randomized clinical trials. *JAMA.* 2017;318:68-81.

57. Katz JN, Zimmerman ZE, Mass H, et al. Diagnosis and management of lumbar spinal stenosis. *JAMA. 2022;327:1688-1699.*

58. Kim TE, Townsend RK, Branch CL, et al. Cannabinoids in the treatment of back pain. *Neurosurgery.* 2020;87:166-175.

59. Komori H, Shinomiya K, Nakai O, et al. The natural history of herniated nucleus pulposus with radiculpathy. *Spine.* 1996;21:225-229.

60. Knezevic NN, Mandalia S, Raasch J, et al. Treatment of chronic low back pain – new approaches on the horizon. *J Pain Res.* 2017;10:1111-1123.

61. Kraychete DC, Sakata RK, Issy AM, et al. Serum cytokine levels in patients with chronic low back pain due to herniated disc: analytical cross-sectional study. *Sao Paulo Med J.* 2010;128:259-262.

62. Lazaro RP, Fenichel GM, Kilroy AW. Congenital muscular dystrophy: case reports and reappraisal. *Muscle and Nerve.* 1979;2:349-355.

63. Lazaro RP. Neuropathic and musculoskeletal pain in carpal tunnel syndrome: prognostic and therapeutic implications. *Surg Neurol.* 1997;47:115-119.

64. Lazaro RP. Electromyography in musculoskeletal pain: a reappraisal and practical considerations. *Surg Neurol Int.* 2015;6:143-146.

65. Lazaro RP. Complex regional pain syndrome: medical and legal ramifications of clinical variability and experience and perspective of a practicing clinician. *J Pain Res.* 2017;10:9-14.

66. Lazaro RP, Butt K. Femoral neuropathy in Lyme Disease. *Int Med Case Rep J.* 2019;12:243-249.

67. Lazaro RP, Eagan TS. A reappraisal of the utility of needle electromyography in low back pain: an observational retrospective study. *Journal of Pain & Relief.* 2020;9(3). doi:10.4172/2167-0846.1000349

68. Lazaro RP. Persistent post-operative low back pain, true radiculopathy and pseudoradiculopathy: retrospective observational study and point of view of a practicing clinician. *Open Journal of Orthopedics.* 2021;11: 289-300.

69. Lazaro RP, Eagan TS. Needle electromyography, F-wave, H-reflex: a critical reappraisal of their utility in the diagnosis of various sensory symptoms in the extremities and spine in the setting of normal neurological examination. *Open Journal of Orthopedics.* 2021;11:383-391.

70. Le Maitre CL, Hoyland JA, Freemont AJ. Catabolic cytokine expression in degenerate and herniated discs: IL-1b and TNFa expression profile. Arthritis Res Ther.2007;9:R77. doi:10.1186/ar2275

71. Lipetz JS. Pathophysiology of inflammatory, degenerative, and compressive radiculopathies. *Phys Med Rehabil Clin N Am.* 2002;13:439-449.

72. Macki M, Hernandez-Hermann M, Bydon M, et al. Spontaneous regression of sequestered lumbar disc herniations: literature review. *Clin Neurol Neurosurg.* 2014;120:136-41.

73. Madden PJ, Lazaro RP. Drooping of the big toe: another diagnostic marker for L5 radiculopathy. *Southern Medical Journal.* 1997;90:209-210.

74. Manchikanti L, Glaser SE, Wolfer L, et al. Systematic review of lumbar discography as a diagnostic test for chronic low back pain. *Pain Physician.* 2009;12:541-559.

75. Marion PJ. Common treatments for low back pain: have they been proven effective? J *Back Musculoskelet Rehabil.* 1995;5:121-133.

76. Maus TP, Bartleson. Diagnosis and therapeutic spinal interventions: Facet Joint. Neurol Clin Pract. 2014;4:342-346.

77. Messiah S, Tharian AR, Candido KD, et al. Neurogenic claudication: a review of current understanding and treatment options. *Curr Pain Headache Rep.* 2019;23(5):32. doi:10.1007/s11916-019-0769

78. Modic MT, Steinberg PM, Ross JS, et al. Degenerative disc disease: assessment of changes in vertebral body marrow with MR imaging. *Radiology.* 1998;166:193-199. doi:10.1148/radiology.166.1.3336678

79. Nakamura SI, Takahashi K, Tkahashi Y, et al. The afferent pathways of discogenic low-back pain. *J Bone Surg* (Br). 1996;78-B:606-612.

80. Nuckley DJ, Kramer PA, Del Rosario A, et al. Intervertebral disc degeneration in a naturally occurring primate model: radiographic and biomechanical evidence. *Journal of Orthopedic Research.* 2008 Sept 26(9):1283-1288. doi:10.1002/jor.20526

81. Oaklander AL, Nolano M. Scientific advances in and clinical approaches to small-fiber polyneuropathy. JAMA Neurol.2019;76:1240-1251. doi:10.1001/jamaneurol 2019.2917

82. Padda M, Khalid K, Zubair U, et al. Stem cell therapy. *Cureus.* 2021;13:e17258. doi:10.7759/cureus.17258

83. Panjabi MM, Goel VK, Takata K. Physiologic strains in the lumbar spinal ligaments: an in vitro biochemical study 1981 Volvo award in biomechanics. *Spine.* 1982;7:192-203. doi:10.1097/00007632-198205000-0003

84. Pomerantz SR. Myelography: modern technique and indications. *Handb Clin Neurol.* 2016;135:193-208.

85. Quattrocchi CC, Alexandre AM, Della Pepa GM, et al. Modic changes: anatomy, pathophysiology and clinical correlation. *Acta Neurochir Suppl.* 2011;108:49-53. doi:10:1007/978-211-99370-5_9

86. Raoul S, Faure A, Rogez JM, et al. Role of sinu-vertebral nerve in low back pain and anatomical basis of therapeutic implications. *Surg Radiol Anat.* 2002;24:366-371.

87. Rea W, Kapur S, Mutagi H. Intervertebral disc as a source of pain. *Continuing Education in Anaesthesia Critical Care.* 2012;12:279-282.

88. Reddi D, Curran. Chronic pain after surgery: pathophysiology, risk factors and prevention. *Postgrad Med.* 2014;90:222-227.

89. Risbud MV, Shapiro IM. Role of cytokine in interverterbral disc degeneration: pain and disc content. *Nature Reviews Rheumatology.* 2013;10:44-56.

90. Ritz BW, Nogusa GM, Perreault MJ, et al. Elevated blood levels of inflammatory monocytes (CD14+ CD 16+) in patients with complex regional pain syndrome. *Clin Exp Immunol.* 2011;164:108-117.

91. Saal AS. Natural history and nonoperative treatment of lumbar disc herniation. *Spine.* 1996;21:254-95.

92. Sanchez-Robles EM, Giron R, Paniagua N, et al. Monoclonal antibodies for chronic pain treatment: present and future. *Int J Mol Sci.* 2021;22(19):10325. doi:10.3390/ijms221910325

93. Sayson JV, Lotz J, Parazynski S, et al. Back pain in space and post-flight spine injury: mechanisms and countermeasure development. *Acat Astronautica.* 2013;86:24-38.

94. Schliessbach J, Siegenthaler A, Heini P, et al. Blockade of the sinuverterbral nerve for the diagnosis of lumbar discogenic pain: an exploratory study. *Anesthesia & Analgesia.* 2010;111:2024-206.

95. Schwarzer AC, Aprill CN, Derby R, et al. The false-positive rate of uncontrolled diagnostic blocks of the lumbar zygapophysial joints. *Pain.* 1994;58:195-200.

96. Schwarzer AC, Aprill CN, Derby R, et al. Clinical features of patients with pain stemming from the lumbar zygapophysial joints. Is the lumbar facet syndrome a clinical entity? *Spine.* 1994;19:1132-1137.

97. Siddall PJ, Cousins MJ. Spine update spinal mechanisms. *Spine.* 1997;22:98-104.

98. Shayota B, Wong TL, Fru D, et al. A comprehensive review of the sinuvertebral nerve with clinical applications. *Anat Cell Biol.* 2019;52:128-133.

99. Shipton EA. Physical therapy approaches in the treatment of low back pain. *Pain Ther.* 2018;7:127-137.

100. Song KJ, Choi BW, Kim GH, et al. Clinical usefulness of CT-myelogram comparing with the MRI in degenerative cervical spinal disorders: is CTM still useful for primary diagnostic tool? *J Spinal Disord Tech.* 2009;22(5):353-357.

101. Sparrey CJ, Bailey JF, Safaee M, et al. Etiology of lumbar lordosis and its pathophysiology: a review of the evolution of lumbar lordosis, and the mechanics and biology of lumbar degeneration. *Journal of Neurosurgery.* 2014;36(5)1-15 doi:103171/2014.1FOCUS13551

102. Staal JB, Nelemans PJ, de Bie BA. Spinal injection therapy for low back pain. *JAMA.* 2013;309:2439-2440.

103. Suseki K, Takahashi Y, Chiba T, et al. Innervation of the lumbar facet joints: origins and functions. *Spine.* 1997;22:477-485.

104. Takahashi H, Suguro T, Okazima Y, et al. Inflammatory cytokines in the herniated disc of the lumbar spine. *Spine.* 1996;21:218-224.

105. Tomkins JP. Alleged human chromosome 2 “Fusion Site” encodes an active DNA binding domain inside a complex and highly expressed gene – negating fusion. *Answers Research Journal.* 2013;6:367-375.

106. Van de Beek WJT, Remarque EJ, Westendorp RGJ, et al. Innate cytokine profile in patients with complex regional pain syndrome is normal. *Pain.* 2001;91:259-262.

107. Van der Heijde D, Dijkmans B, Geusens P, et al. Efficacy and safety of infliximab in patients with ankylosing spondylitis: results of a randomized, placebo-controlled trial (ASSERT). *Arthritis Rheum.* 2009;52:582-591.

108. Van Poppel MNM, Koes BW, Van der Ploeg T, et al. Lumbar supports and education for the prevention of low back pain. *JAMA.* 1998;279:1789-1794.

109. Van Tulder MW, Assendelft WJJ, Koes BW, et al. Spinal radiographic findings and nonspecific low back pain. *Spine.* 1997;22:427-434.

110. Weber KT, Alipui DO, Sison CP, et al. Serum levels of the proinflammatory cytokine interleukin-6 vary based on diagnoses in individuals with lumbar intervertebral disc diseases. *Arthritis Research & Therapy.* 2016;18:3. doi:10.1186/s13075-015-0887-8

111. Weglinski MR, Wedek, Engel AG. Malignant hyperthermia testing in patients with persistently increased serum creatine kinase levels. *Anesth Anal.* 1997;84:1038-1041.

112. Won HS, Yang M, Kim YD. Facet joint injections for management of low back pain: a clinically focused review. *Anesth Pain Med.* 2020;15:8-18.

113. Wright MH, Denney LC. A comprehensive review of spinal arachnoiditis. *Ortho Nurs.* 2003;22:215-219.

114. Wu J, Du Z, Lv Y, et al. A new technique for the treatment of lumbar facet joint syndrome using intra-articular injection with autologous rich plasma. *Pain Physician.* 2016;19:617-625.

115. Wuertz K, Haglund L. Inflammatory mediators in intervertebral disc degeneration and discogenic pain. Global Spine J. 2013;3:175-184.

116. Xiaogang M, Quanshan H, Liping Z, et al. The expression of cytokine and its significance for the intervertebral discs of Kazakhs. *J Clin Lab Anal.* 2016;31(5):e22087.

117. Zeng ZF, Liang YR, Chen Y, et al. Chronic back pain cured by low-dose levodopa: is it a variant of restless legs syndrome. *J Pain Res.* 2018;11:277-279.

118. Zhang JM, An J. Cytokines, inflammation, and pain. *Int Anesthesiol Clin.* 2007;45:27-37.

119. Zhang Q, Cheng K, Yan H, et al. The anatomical study and clinical significance of the sinuvertebral nerves at the lumbar levels. *Spine.* 2020;45(2):e61-e66. doi:10.1097/BRS.0000000000003190

120. Zhang YH, Zhao CQ, Jiang LS, et al. Modic changes: a systematic review of the literature. *Eur Spine J.* 2008;17:1289-129. doi:10:10.1007/s00586-008-0758-y

BOOKS

1. Ropper AH, Samuels MA. *Adams and Victor's Principles of Neurology*. 9th ed. McGraw Hill; 2009.

2. Drake RL, Vogl W, Mitchell AWM. *Gray's Anatomy for students*. Elsevier; 2005:69-70

3. Jorde LB, Carey JC, Bamshad MJ. *Medical Genetics*. Elsevier; 2019.

4. Hart W. *The Genesis Race*. Bear and Company; 2003.

5. Adams F. *Origins of Existence*. The Free Press; 2002.

6. Alshak MN, Das JM. *Neuroanatomy, Sympathetic Nervous System*. StatPearls Publishing; 2022.

7. Brooke MH. *A Clinicians View of Neuromusular Disorders*, 2nd ed. Williams and Wilkins; 1986.

8. Fenichel GM. *Neonatal Neurology*. Churchill Livingstone; 1980.

ONLINE SOURCES

1. Blood supply of the lumbar spine - Radiology Key - radiologykey.com-supply-of-the-lumbar-spine
2. The sympathetic nerves - Human Anatomy – Theodora.com/anatomy/the _sympathetic _ nerves.html
3. New Research Debunks Human Chromosome Fusion – www.icr.org/article/new-research-debunks-human
4. Debunking the Debunkers/Answers Research Journal – answersresearchjournal.org/debunking-the –debunkers
5. Human and chimp DNA: Is it Really 98% similar? – genesisapologetics.com/faqs/human-and-chimp-dna
6. Proof Humans Didn't Evolve from Apes – The Truth Source – the truthsource.org/proof-humans-didn't-evolve
7. Lumbar discography. Position statement from the North American Spine Society – pubmed.ncbi.nlm.nih.gov/8578384
8. Frequency of Epidural Steroid Injections – cdn.ymaws.com/www.spineintervention.org
9. Non-operative management: An evidence-based approach – www.sciencedirect.com/science
10. Complications of Spinal Cord Stimulation – www.asra.com/guidelines-articles/original
11. Spinal Cord Stimulator/Johns Hopkins Medicine – www.hopkinsmedicine.org/health/treatment
12. Gadolinium-based contrast agent toxicity – www.ncbi.nih/pmc/articles/PMC4879157
13. What is clinical thermography? – spinalalignment.com/thermography-pain-management
14. Thermography in the diagnosis of low back pain – www.sciencedirect.com/science/article
15. Thermography in low back pain and sciatica – pubmed.ncbi.nih.gov/2931061
16. Medical Infrared Thermography in back pain – pubmed.ncbi.nlm.nih.gov/30012388
17. Anti-IL-17 monoclonal antibodies for the treatment of ankylosing spondylitis – pubmed-ncbi.nlm.nih.gov/30500270
18. Post-Flight Back Pain Following International Space Station Missions: Evaluation of Spaceflight Risk Factors – ntrs.nasa.gov/api/citations/20150020953
19. Upright positional MRI of the lumbar spine – PubMed – pubmed.ncbi.nlm.gov/18718234
20. Injectable gel shows promise as treatment for back pain – www.painnewsnetwork.org/stories/2022
21. A new injectable gel may greatly reduce chronic low back pain – neurosciencenews.com/hydrogel-back-pain-20785
22. Low Back Pain Exercises – MC7245-464 – Mayo Clinic Health System - www.mayoclinichealthsystem.org
23. Small fiber neuropathy associated with SARS-CoV-2 infection – www.ncbi.nlm.nih.gov/pmc/articles

24, Fibromyalgia and small fiber neuropathy: the plot thickens – pubmed.ncbi.nlm.nih.gov/3023832

25. Small fiber neuropathy as a part of fibromyalgia or a separate diagnosis – www.openaccessjournals.com/articles/smallfiber

26, How Best to Diagnose Small Fiber Neuropathy: Neurology Today – journals.lww.com/neurotodayonline/fulltext/2019

27. Stem cell therapy in discogenic back pain – www.ncbi.nlm.nih.gov/pmc/article/PMC /6989932

28. Intracept Procedure for Chronic Lower Back Pain Relief – www.sciatica.com/treatment/intracept-procedure
29. Basivertebral Nerve Ablation-PubMed – pubmed.ncbi.nlm.nih.gov/34283493
30. Basivertebral Nerve Ablation – StatPearls – NCBI – www.ncbi.nlm.nih.gov/books/NBK/572127
31. Nanotechnology Back Research – wexnermedical.osu.edu
32. Nanotechnology: A Promising New Paradigm for the Control of Pain – academic.oup.com/painmedicine/article.19/2/232
33. Spinal injections with imaging guidance –Choosing Wisely – www.choosingwisely.org/clinician-lists/north
34. North American Spine Society – Choosing Wisely – www.choosingwisely.org/societies/north-american

FIGURE LEGENDS **(art works provided by Maa Illustrations, art@maaillustrations.com)**

1. Lateral view of the lumbar spine showing the intervertebral disks and the magnified view of the two vertebrae and the disk in between. The facet joints (or zygapophyseal joints), when they become inflamed, generate LBP. The structure behind the disk pointing obliquely and downward is the spinal nerve root, which, when compressed by the herniated disk, can lead to radicular pain or numbness in the corresponding dermatome along with focal muscle weakness, such as foot drop.

2. Cross-section of the vertebra above the termination of the spinal cord. The spinal nerve is formed from the union between the dorsal and ventral roots. The sinuvertebral nerve arises from the ventral ramus and innervates the disks (vertical yellow lines). It contains sympathetic nerve fibers originating from the sympathetic chain, which interconnect with the vertebra above and below. The presence of sympathetic fibers will explain the various autonomic symptoms in the lower extremities experienced by most patients with discogenic pain.

3. Lateral view of the arterial supply of the lumbar spine. pscb: posterior spinal canal branch, dr: branch to dorsal ramus, vr: branch to ventral ramus, ia: branch to pars articularis, ascb: anterior spinal canal branch, LA: lumbar artery, man: metaphyseal anastomosis, ppa: primary periosteal artery, spa: secondary periosteal artery, ana: anastomosis over the disk.

4. These are the sensory dermatomes; each territory corresponds to sensory root innervation. Symptoms consist of a numb or tingly (or both) sensation over the sensory territory.

5. Diagrammatic representation of a herniated lumbar disk and inflammation of surrounding structures (red shading).

6. Lumbar herniated disk demonstrated by MRI (encircled broad red arrow). The disk above showed early signs of degeneration (loss of whitish hue compared to the prominent whitish hue in the intervertebral disks above it).

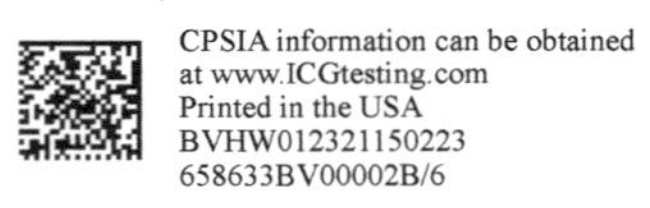

CPSIA information can be obtained
at www.ICGtesting.com
Printed in the USA
BVHW012321150223
658633BV00002B/6